ANALYSIS OF PERCEPTION

Founded by C. K. Ogden

The International Library of Psychology

COGNITIVE PSYCHOLOGY
In 21 Volumes

ANALYSIS OF PERCEPTION

J R SMYTHIES

Preface by Sir Russell Brain

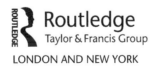

Routledge
Taylor & Francis Group
LONDON AND NEW YORK

First published in 1956 by
Routledge
2 Park Square, Milton Park, Abingdon, Oxfordshire OX14 4RN
711 Third Avenue, New York, NY 10017

First issued in paperback 2014

Routledge is an imprint of the Taylor and Francis Group, an informa business

British Library Cataloguing in Publication Data
A CIP catalogue record for this book
is available from the British Library

Analysis of Perception
ISBN 0415-20974-9
Cognitive Psychology: 21 Volumes
ISBN 0415-21126-3
The International Library of Psychology: 204 Volumes
ISBN 0415-19132-7

ISBN 13: 978-1-138-87507-4 (pbk)
ISBN 13: 978-0-415-20974-8 (hbk)

CONTENTS

PREFACE

FOR many years it has been known that perception depends in some way upon the brain, but until recently so little was known about the brain that philosophers who wrote about perception could confine themselves to a linguistic exposition of their own introspection and a time-worn stock-in-trade of illusions and hallucinations, such as pink rats, of which they had usually no personal experience. During the last twenty-five years, however, such large additions have been made to the neurophysiology of perception that philosophers can no longer afford to neglect this aspect of their subject. Unfortunately, like other developments of science, this new knowledge is highly technical. The philosopher who would do justice to perception today must have in addition to his philosophical training an advanced knowledge of neurophysiology, electronics, neurology, psychology and psychiatry, and preferably should himself have taken a hallucinogenic drug. Probably no single person is thus fully equipped, but Dr. Smythies possesses an exceptional range of knowledge in these fields, and this has enabled him to make what is so far a unique contribution to our knowledge of perception. He takes a representationalist view, and it is difficult to see what alternative can survive an acquaintance not merely with the distortions of perception caused by disease of the brain and the rich variety of hallucinatory experiences, but even with the analysis of normal perception produced by the stroboscope. He disposes of the theory of projected sensations, and adopting Bertrand Russell's idea of physical and perceptual worlds, proceeds to discuss the possible geometries of their mutual relations. Here he is wisely tentative.

The value of this book is that the author has made available to students of philosophy much new knowledge of the first importance. He has opened a door through which many may enter and go where their own thinking leads them.

RUSSELL BRAIN.

vii

INTRODUCTION

IN an era of ever-increasing specialisation it becomes difficult to keep sight of one of the proper tasks of philosophy—that defined by Broad as the synopsis and synthesis of the various branches of knowledge. In the last few decades there have been great advances in, for example, physics, chemistry and biochemistry, neuroanatomy and neurophysiology, linguistics and mathematical logic and it has become very difficult, as Brain has pointed out, for any one man to have expert knowledge of more than one of these fields of study. Workers in each specialty make progress but 'no one is capable of creating a synthesis or discovering relations between the facts discovered by the various specialists; indeed, the very facts themselves are often unknown to the philosophers. What then is to be done?'[1] In order to construct a comprehensive theory of perception, or to give an exhaustive account of the mind and its place in nature, it would be necessary to have at least a good working knowledge of the following subjects: epistemology and the philosophy of sense-perception, neurology, neuroanatomy and neurophysiology, psychiatry and psychopathology with particular reference to the effects produced by the hallucinogenic drugs, anthropology, physics and experimental psychology. Philosophy has become itself one of the specialties, and no philosopher has, so far as I know, set out to gain such a working knowledge of these subjects as a basis for his philosophising. A philosopher turned specialist (e.g. a specialist in the 'logical analysis of language') may be able to give an account of perception adequate from his own limited standpoint. Inadequacies of his account may only become apparent when we evaluate it against the factual evidence contained in one of the other specialties. I cannot accept

[1] Sir Russell Brain (a), *Mind, Perception and Science*, Oxford, 1951, p. 3.

Introduction

the view that an adequate and comprehensive account of perception can be given solely in terms of an analysis of ordinary language. A study of the perceptual processes themselves is obligatory. Neurobiological theorists themselves have not been concerned with the fundamental problems of sense-perception and epistemology. Their attention has largely been taken up with the limited problems of their own specialty. At most attempts have been made to analyse the basic concepts of one specialty in terms of another higher on the positivistic hierarchy —e.g. Hebb's attempt to base learning theory on neurophysiological principles[1] and Köhler's more ambitious attempt to link Gestalt theory with field theories in physics.[2] As far as I know only Brain has made an attempt to correlate modern neurology and epistemology.[3]

There are in particular two such major fields of study on perception between which there has been, as yet, very little liaison. The first consists of the analytical work of certain English philosophers—notably Broad, Price and Earl Russell—into the nature of the perceptual process. The second comprises the studies made over the last fifty years—largely by German neurologists—on the changes produced in perception by brain injuries and disease, by certain chemical agents such as mescaline and by physical agents such as the electronic stroboscope. Now if one studies both these fields at once it becomes clear that:

(1) The philosophers construct their arguments neglecting most of this evidence from neurology which must surely be of crucial importance in any comprehensive account of perception. For instance, many philosophers bring in the argument from illusion and hallucination at some point in their analysis of perception. In this they are content to give a few instances of hallucinatory sense-experiences—usually the 'pink rats' of the alcoholic—and, in general, they do not prepare for their epistemological analysis by first making a thorough study of hallucinations themselves. This can lead to unfortunate results.[4] In

[1] D. O. Hebb, *The Organisation of Behaviour*, New York, 1949.
[2] Wolfgang Köhler in *Cerebral Mechanisms in Behavior. The Hixon Symposium*, New York, 1951, p. 200 and elsewhere.
[3] Brain, loc. cit. (*a*).
[4] J. R. Smythies (*a*), 'A note on Mr. Hirst's recent paper in Mind', *Mind*, 1954, **63**, 388–9.

any case it could be claimed that a wider acquaintance with the nature of hallucinatory sense-experience and its relation to veridical sense-experience will give our epistemological theories a sounder basis.

(2) The neurologists present their facts and theories in terms which are often somewhat confused and much in need of a critical philosophical analysis. The same terms may be used to refer to a number of different processes and entities. The epistemological position at the basis of contemporary neurology is also unsatisfactory in that incompatible theories of perception are entertained simultaneously. This muddle gives rise to the need to invent a number of pseudo-processes, such as the alleged 'projection' of sensations, for the actual existence of which no evidence has been found. The origins, extent and cure for these muddles are analysed below.

I will not be concerned in this book with a choice between rival *philosophical* theories of perception, but I will attempt to show that, if a comprehensive scientific theory of perception can be constructed, then the philosophical puzzles about perception—together with the purely philosophical theories evoked by these puzzles—will, as it were, wither away. Such a comprehensive scientific theory of perception will explain just *how* our raw sensory experience is related to the physiological process of perception and, in doing this, it will automatically take care of such philosophical puzzles as 'where are sense-data?', 'what are the relations between sense-data and physical things; or between sense-data and the brain?', etc. It will be clear that the theory here to be presented has been developed out of the traditional representative theory, but it differs from this in several important respects which will receive comment.

In Chapter 1 I make a logical analysis of the relation between sensory experience and the physical and physiological processes of perception. The neurological evidence is presented in Chapter 2. Chapter 3 is devoted to a discussion of the neurological concept of the body-image, the confusion over which has befogged a quantity of invaluable neurological evidence relevant to the epistemological status of sense-data. In Chapter 4 I present an account of hallucinatory sense-experience with particular reference to Ayer's analysis. The last two chapters give discussions, somewhat aside from the main argument contained in the first four chapters, of Price's analysis of perception and of Sherrington's analysis of mind. Finally a brief account is given of possible ways in which these new theories of perception may be verified by experiment.

I shall use the symbols ⟨ ⟩ enclosing a word to indicate that I am talking about the word itself. The symbols ' ' enclosing a sentence indicate a statement or a quotation and around a phrase or single word indicate either a quotation or that some special, unusual, doubtful or questionable use of the phrase or word is entailed. All lettered superscripts refer to the additional notes at the end of the book.

I am most grateful to Sir Russell Brain, Professor H. H. Price and Dr. R. H. Thouless for their help and advice. The final form of this work owes much to conversation with Professor A. G. N. Flew, Mrs. Martha Kneale and Professor C. W. K. Mundle at Le Piol, St. Paul-de-Vence in April 1954, and with Professor Peter Remnant and Professor Avrum Stroll at the University of British Columbia and with Mr. B. S. Benjamin at the Australian National University. Mrs. Cheyney, Medical Artist at the University of British Columbia, very kindly drew the figures. I am grateful to the Editor of *The British Journal for the Philosophy of Science* for permission to reproduce material from the following papers appearing in the journal: 'The Mescaline Phenomena'; 'Analysis of Projection'; and 'An Empirical Verification of the Representative Theory of Perception'.[a] I should also like to take this opportunity to thank Captain Alfred Hubbard of Long Beach, California, whose generosity made it possible to complete this work, and to record my gratitude to my colleagues in research—Professor Abram Hoffer, Edward Osborn Esq. and Dr. Humphrey Osmond—who have aided me in so many ways that I will always be in their debt. The main part of this book was completed during the tenure of part of a Nuffield Fellowship in Medicine in the Department of Physiology, Australian National University.

THE PSYCHOLOGICAL LABORATORY,
DOWNING STREET,
CAMBRIDGE.

PROLOGUE

THIS sharp division between the clarity of finite science and the dark universe beyond is itself an abstraction from concrete fact. For example, we can explore our presuppositions. Take the special case of natural science, we presuppose geometry. But what sort of geometry? There are many kinds. In fact, there are an indefinite number of alternative geometries. Which one are we to choose?

We all know that this is a topic which has bothered, or elated, physical science during the last thirty years. At last the great scientists are coming to conclusions which we will all accept. And yet a sceptical doubt intrudes. How do we know that only one geometry is relevant to the complex happenings of nature? Perhaps a three-dimensional geometry is relevant to one sort of occurrences; and a fifteen-dimensional geometry is required for another sort. . . .

Perhaps our knowledge is distorted unless we can comprehend its essential connection with happenings which involve spatial relationships of fifteen dimensions. The dogmatic assumption of the trinity of nature as its sole important dimensional aspect has been useful in the past. It is becoming dangerous in the present. In the future it may be a fatal barrier to the advance of knowledge.

Also, this planet, or this nebula in which our sun is placed, may be gradually advancing towards a change in the general character of its spatial relations. Perhaps in the dim future mankind, if it then exists, will look back to the queer, contracted three-dimensional universe from which the nobler, wider existence has emerged.

These speculations are, at present, neither proved nor disproved. They have however a mythical value. They do represent how concentration on coherent verbalisations of certain aspects of human experience may block the advance of understanding. Too many apples from the tree of systemised knowledge lead to the fall of progress.

ALFRED NORTH WHITEHEAD from *Modes of Thought*
(Cambridge, 1938, pp. 77–9)

Chapter One

THE REPRESENTATIVE
THEORY OF PERCEPTION

1.　MY main purpose in this book is to construct the outline of a comprehensive neurological theory of perception. A neurological theory of perception may either be 'local'—that is concerned only with the detail of events in one or other part of the nervous system—or it may be a theory designed to give a comprehensive account of all the processes that mediate perception. The main task before such a comprehensive theory at present is to give an account of the relation between our sensory experience and the physical and physiological processes of perception. This problem is closely allied to two other unsolved problems of neurology: that of the nature of 'consciousness' and that of the mind-brain relation. In spite of all the enquiry and analysis that have been directed at these problems in recent years—by philosophers, psychologists and neurologists—no generally acceptable solution has been reached. I shall argue that the reason for these continued failures has not lain in any fatal difficulty in the problems themselves; nor can we call them 'pseudo-problems' for which no real answers are logically attainable. The attempts have failed for two main reasons: (*a*) the basic terms in the theories have not been adequately defined, and no adequate criteria have been given to determine what it is exactly that the terms used in these theories refer; and (*b*) elements that should have been taken into account have been omitted.

1.1.   These problems belong to both philosophy and science. Yet philosophers interested in perception have not concerned themselves to any great extent with the relation between sense-experience and the physiological processes of perception. They have concerned themselves instead very largely with epistemological questions. The problem of perception has been seen as a *logical* problem about the logical status of our knowledge of the external world.[1] These philosophers have debated questions such as how this knowledge may legitimately be based on 'an acquaintance with sense-data', or whether statements about physical objects can be reduced to statements about sense-data, etc. The methods used in these investigations have usually consisted of a careful analysis of the philosopher's own normal perception in an attempt to discover what exactly is occurring in perceptual situations, and of purely linguistic or logical analyses of statements that could be made in various perceptual situations. It can be argued, however, that these methods are inadequate to give us a comprehensive and valid theory of perception. Russell[2] has already dealt with the claim put forward by some members of the linguistic school that an analysis of ordinary language is sufficient to settle all philosophical disputes (and see also Chapter 4). Furthermore important phenomena (e.g. the stroboscopic phenomena, see Chapter 2) that are necessary to our understanding of perception are, in fact, inaccessible to normal perception, and they can only be revealed by using special methods, or by studying perception in unusual or pathological states of the nervous system. To give another example, some philosophers are prepared to write at length about hallucinations without ever having made a close study of these phenomena, either by reading the extensive psychopathological literature, or by talking to people who are having or who have had hallucinations, or, best of all, by having some hallucinations for themselves. They thus depend on common hearsay or folk

[1] See A. M. Quinton, 'The problem of perception', *Mind*, 1955, **64**, 28–51.
[2] Lord Russell (*a*), 'The cult of common-usage', *Brit. J. Phil. Sci.*, 1953, **3**, 303–7.

beliefs for their sources of information. Few contemporary philosophers appear to consider that physiology or neurology could contribute to the solution of fundamental problems of perception and mind-brain relation.

Those philosophers (such as Lord Russell and Professor Broad) who have paid most attention to the physiological account of perception have usually held some form of the sense-datum theory, but this theory has never been able to give an unambiguous definition of the central term of the theory ⟨sense-datum⟩, nor has it been able to give any very clear account of the relation between sense-data and physical objects. For this and other reasons[1] the theory has fallen into considerable disfavour amongst contemporary philosophers, who claim that there are no such entities as sense-data to mediate our perception of the external world, but that what sense-datum theorists would like to call ⟨sense-data⟩ *really are* physical objects or, at any rate, parts of physical objects. Most contemporary philosophers would support some form of naïve realism (see the writings of Ryle, Ayer, Warnock, Hirst, Quinton, Lean, etc.).

1.2. Now the evidence from physics, physiology and neurology has clearly demonstrated that the causal processes of perception (i.e. in the case of vision the causal chain: physical object—light—retina—optic nerve—central nervous system) are a necessary condition for any (veridical) perception to occur.

---

[1] It has been held that the 'argument from illusion' and the scientific account of perception both show that we could not be directly aware of (or directly experience) external physical objects, but that we are directly aware of (or directly experience) something else called ⟨sense-data⟩ or ⟨sensa⟩. It was further held (i) that only statements about sense-data could be certainly true (excluding deliberate lying and slips of the tongue as well as all analytical statements and tautologies) whereas statements about physical objects could only be to various degrees probable and never certainly true (owing to the ever-present possibility of illusion and hallucination phenomenologically indistinguishable from veridical perception); and (ii) that our knowledge about physical objects is derived by a species of inference from our knowledge of sense-data. Quinton (loc. cit.) argues that both these beliefs are mistaken because (i) statements about sense-data are no more certainly true than are statements about physical objects and (ii) because no species of inference is involved in our direct perception of physical objects.

But there have been differences of opinion amongst neurologists about what the last term in this causal chain should be and about the relation of the perception itself to this chain. The monist school has held that this causal chain leads from the primary sensory cortex to other parts of the brain and finally to the motor cortex, and so movements of the body are produced. The causal chain is confined by this school entirely to the physical world. The dualist school extends this causal chain by one more term on its afferent side, and postulates that the cerebral events bear a causal relation to events external to the brain. That is to say it is postulated that certain cerebral events cause a 'sensation' (or 'impression', 'conscious experience', etc.) to arise in the 'mind' (or in 'consciousness', 'direct awareness', etc.). The motor cortex is then supposed to be influenced directly by the 'mind' ('consciousness', etc.) as well as by other parts of the brain including the sensory areas. Thus the monist causal chain of perception and action reads:

receptor organ—nervous system—effector organ

The dualist causal chain reads:

receptor organ—nervous system—mind—nervous system—

effector organ.

(The dotted line indicates the path taken by the causal processes mediating the control of automatic movements or the automatic component of voluntary movements.) The left half of the dualist chain is the chain of perception and the right half is the chain of voluntary movement. Neither theory has been able to give a coherent account of the relation between this causal chain and the perception itself except to say that the former is a necessary condition for the latter to occur. Moreover, the dualist theory has been handicapped for the same reason that the sense-datum theory in philosophy has been abandoned by so many philosophers; and that is a fatal lack of rigid definition of its basic terms. I shall argue that a synthesis of the sense-datum theory with the neurological account of perception may constitute, if its basic terms can receive adequate definition, the only valid theory of perception in both science and philosophy, for, as I will attempt to demonstrate, it is the only theory that

4

does not lead to logical fallacies when conjoined with certain well-established scientific facts. It may well be that the reasons that some philosophers have given for holding the sense-datum theory are invalid, and yet the sense-datum theory itself, in some form, may be correct.[b]

2. In order to give a satisfactory account of perception we must define the basic terms to be used as rigidly as possible, and we must take care that all the events concerned in the perception are described in the theory. Similarly in order to give an account of the relation between experiential events and brain events (and between sense-data and the brain), we must first (2.1) delineate exactly what experiential events *are* and how to recognise them, and then (2.2) we must determine what features they possess which will enable us to *relate* them to brain events. To consider these in turn:

2.1. I will first define the basic terms to be used in this theory.
Definition 1. *Sense-datum*. Warnock[1] has pointed out that the word ⟨sense-datum⟩ 'like the word "idea" in Berkeley's time, has by now been so frequently *used* that many people seem merely to take for granted that its meaning is clear and well understood; though enquiry would show that this is very far from being the case'. Russell's original definition of ⟨sense-datum⟩ ran as follows[2]: '. . . the things that are immediately known in sensation: such things as colours, sounds, smells, hardnesses, roughnesses, and so on.' Broad[3] gives the name ⟨sensa⟩ to 'the objective constituents of perceptual situations . . .[4] Under certain conditions I have states of mind called sensations. These sensations have objects, which are always concrete particular existents, like coloured or hot patches, noises, smells etc. Such objects are called sensa.' Moore[5] has used the term to denote 'whatever is directly perceived in sensory experience'. Now Quinton[6] has recently drawn attention to

---

[1] G. J. Warnock, *Berkeley*, Pelican edition, p. 237.
[2] Lord Russell (*b*), *The Problems of Philosophy*, London, 1912, p. 17.
[3] C. D. Broad (*a*), *The Mind and its Place in Nature*, London, 1925, p. 182.
[4] C. D. Broad (*b*), *Scientific Thought*, London, 1923, p. 243.
[5] G. E. Moore, quoted by Martin Lean, *Sense-Perception and Matter*, London, 1953, p. 7.
[6] Quinton, loc. cit.

the difficulties of defining ⟨sense-datum⟩ in terms of so difficult a concept as 'direct experience'. Furthermore a definition of ⟨sense-datum⟩ clearly will not do if it can be used to refer to physical objects as well. Yet every term used by Russell and Broad to exemplify sense-data is taken from common-usage, where it ordinarily refers to physical objects or parts of physical objects. For example, ⟨coloured patch⟩ may be used to describe parts of a painting or a person's cheek. One can meaningfully talk of the sound of a waterfall in the wilderness never visited by man, the smell of a fox near the waterfall, of lichens forming coloured patches on stones in the vicinity and so on. If these terms can be used where no sensation is implied their use as *definitions* of the elements of sensation would be confusing to say the least. A phenomenalist would claim that the examples I have given are instances of 'potential' sense-data. But to this we can reply that we require an unambiguous definition of actual sense-data. Furthermore we need a definition that applies to sense-data only, and that will be valid whatever theory of perception is correct.

It is, however, possible to give a definition of ⟨sense-datum⟩ in terms not of a dubious relation to undefined terms such as ⟨direct experience⟩, or to physical objects, or to words such as ⟨sound⟩, ⟨colour patch⟩, etc., but in terms of an observed relationship to such familiar phenomena as after-sensations, which need no formal definitions themselves; for they can receive adequate *ostensive* and *operational* definitions. We can instruct anyone how to set about observing an after-sensation, and no one is likely to confuse an after-sensation with a physical object. The reader is now invited to perform the following experiment. Obtain an after-sensation by looking at a single frosted electric lamp bulb of some 60-watt power and conventional shape from a distance of three feet away for about five seconds, and then look away. If you can observe the following spatial relations of the after-sensation you will be able to use definition 1.1. which states:

Definition 1.1. 'If the boundary J of the after-sensation (hereafter *y*) can be observed to describe a Jordan curve in the total field composed of *x* and *y* such that it divides this total field into one *inside* and one *outside*, then *x* is a sense-datum.'

In more technical terms this may be put as follows:

Definition 1.2. 'If the boundary J of y can be observed to form a Jordan curve which decomposes $x + y - J$ into two regions whose common boundary is J, then x is a sense-datum.' And in *definiendum-definiens* form:

Definition 1.3. 'A sense-datum is a spatial entity that may be so spatially related to an after-sensation (y) that the boundary J of y decomposes (the spatial entity $+ y - J$) into two regions whose common boundary is J.'

In the case of those sense-data that occupy a smaller proportion of the total visual field than is occupied by y, empirical observation will show that the following modification of our definition will be necessary:

Definition 1.4. 'If the boundary J' of x forms a Jordan curve which decomposes $y + x - J'$ into two regions whose common boundary is J', then x is a sense-datum.'

It may however be objected that after-sensations are not exactly spatially inside sense-data as a circle in a plane may be said to be inside the plane, but that the after-sensation is a little nearer the observer than is the sense-datum. Anyone can investigate this matter by observing his own after-sensations and their relations to his own sense-data. To answer this objection we can amend our original definition in one of two ways:

Definition 2. 'If the *geometrical projection* of y on x has a boundary J which describes a Jordan curve that decomposes $x - J$ into two regions whose common boundary is J, then x is a sense-datum.'

Definition 3. 'If a part of x can be covered by y in such a way that the part of x covered by y has a boundary J that describes a Jordan curve . . . (continued as in definition 2).' A variation based on the concepts of Gestalt psychology may be constructed as follows:

Definition[1] 4. 'Any x is a sense-datum if it can be observed

---

[1] All these 'definitions', except 1.3, may perhaps more accurately be regarded as *criteria* for discovering sense-data or for finding out what are to be named sense-data rather than *strict logical definitions* of the term ⟨sense-datum⟩ of which 1.3 may be the only example in the collection. But this may be a debatable point. In any case such criteria will meet our requirements. Note also that Definition 1.3 may be modified in the same way, *mutatis mutandis*, as Definitions 1.4, 2 and 3 were modified with respect to Definition 1.2.

to bear the relationship of forming a *ground* to the *figure* formed by *y*.' This employs the figure-ground relationship of Gestalt psychology. (Definitions 2–4 may be modified in the same way, *mutatis mutandis*, as Definition 1.4 was modified with respect to Definition 1.2.)

Similar definitions can be constructed for tactual sense-data in terms of their observed spatial relations to tactual after-sensations. For instance, we can press on the skin with three rods placed in a straight line. If we then remove the outer couple, we could define the tactual sense-datum 'as that which was felt to be spatially between the two tactual after-sensations experienced'. But clearly this method will not work as elegantly in the case of tactual sense-data as it does in the case of visual sense-data, and it will not work at all in the case of non-extended sense-data, such as auditory, olfactory and gustatory ones, which have the further defect (from our present point of view) in that they have very ill-defined after-sensations.

These definitions or criteria will not however be suitable in the following cases: (2.11) those sense-data related to objects fleetingly glimpsed—for there will be no time to carry out the test; and (2.12) those related to a large number of objects seen simultaneously—for by the time that the test has been carried out on the first members of the group it may be that those sense-data that were related to the other members of the group of physical objects might have been replaced by other sense-data related to these objects. How then can we extend our criteria to cover these cases? For clearly the criteria should be applicable to all sense-data and not merely to a few. There may not be any reasonable doubt that if, in (2.11), we had been able to get an after-sensation quickly enough we would have been able to observe that it did in fact bear the required relation to the sense-data momentarily sensed; or, in (2.12), that we could rightly say, 'If I had placed my after-sensation in all those other sense-data then I could have observed the required relation.' But such conditional statements cannot qualify as rigid criteria for determining what are to be named sense-data. In order to cover these special cases we can identify a suitable 'standard' sense-datum *x* in any visual field by using the criteria listed above, and then we can identify all other sense-data in the field by saying 'if any χ is observed to be sensibly contiguous with x or with another χ, then χ is a sense-datum'. We can define ⟨sensibly contiguous⟩ in this context by saying that x and χ both have boundaries and if part of the boundary of x is identical with part of the boundary of χ then x and χ are sensibly contiguous.

Definition 5. *Sensing.* This term may be defined as the relation between an observer (I or Pure Ego) and a sense-datum in any perception. However some philosophers (notably Hume) have denied the existence of any such entity as a Pure Ego. Furthermore it seems impossible to give any rigid definition of the term. So we can, if pressed, dispense with it altogether if sense-data are simply held to *occur* in conjunction with certain images, thoughts, feelings, attitudes, sets of attention, etc. In which case the statement 'I sensed a sense-datum' will be equivalent to the statement 'a certain sense-datum occurred in such and such circumstances'. Similarly the term ⟨sense-experience⟩ will be equivalent to the term ⟨the occurrence of a sense-datum⟩. It will be convenient to distinguish between *sensing* sense-data and *examining* sense-data. Although this analysis of perception shows that sense-data do enter into all perceptions, most people do not consider this in their normal everyday occupations and usually regard themselves simply as seeing houses, people, clouds, stars, etc. In such a case I will say that 'sensing' is the relation between an observer and a sense-datum when the person is simply about his daily business and considers himself simply to be seeing physical objects. However, as soon as a philosopher or psychologist has distinguished entities in his visual field which he names ⟨sense-data⟩, he can examine these, as it were, in themselves without necessary reference to physical objects. This deliberate philosophical examination of a sense-datum may be called 'examining a sense-datum'. The perceptual processes in each case are the same; only the psychological attitude, purpose and descriptive vocabulary of the person are different. Quinton refers to the special 'phenomenological' frame of mind in which what I call examining a sense-datum is carried out.

Definition 6. *Experiential event.* Sense-data are not merely static entities but may be observed to move (i.e. to change their

9

position in the visual field), to change their shape, to swell and shrink, and in general to *change*.

'The distinction between *fixed* and *moving* sense-data is a qualitative contrast directly perceived. It cannot therefore be defined. The distinction can only be indicated by means of expressions which contain it. A datum is fixed if it retains a constant extension or the same position in the sense field during its whole duration. On the other hand, a datum is moving if its extension varies in the course of its duration, either by deformation or by displacement.'[1]

So we can define an *experiential event* as any change in any sense-datum or any replacement of any one sense-datum by another.

Definition 7. *Visual field.* The visual field of any individual human being may be defined as the totality of visual sense-data sensed by that individual during any specious present. Similarly the somatic sensory field may be defined as the totality of somatic sense-data sensed by the individual during any specious present.

2.2. I will next list a series of empirical facts about sense-data so that we may discover how best to relate sense-data to a brain.

2.21. A sense-datum is a spatial entity. As Ayer says,[2] 'The extension and figure of a visual sense-datum are sensibly "given" no less than its colour; . . .' (If we use Definition 1.3 this becomes an analytical statement.)

2.22. Sense-data bear *spatial relations* to other sense-data. Among these relations may be discerned the following:

2.221. Sense-data may be *inside* or *outside* other sense-data in a topological sense. For instance, the sense-datum related to the yolk of a fried egg looked at from above is topologically inside the sense-datum related to the white of the egg. In general sense-data may be said to satisfy many of the axioms and theorems of topology.

2.222. Two sense-data may share, in part, a common boundary —i.e. they may be contiguous. Or other sense-data may wholly

[1] Jean Nicod, *Foundations of Geometry and Induction*, London, 1930, p. 54.
[2] A. J. Ayer, *The Foundations of Empirical Knowledge*, New York, 1940, p. 246.

separate them in which case they may be said to be non-contiguous.

2.223. Every sense-datum is contiguous with at least one other sense-datum (except in the case where the whole visual field is filled with one entirely uniform sense-datum).

2.224. Sense-data are contiguous at every portion of their boundaries with other sense-data. The only exceptions to this rule are those sense-data at the extreme periphery of the visual field and possibly those bordering on the 'blind spot'.

2.225. *Some* sense-data, e.g. those related to stars, may be held to be 'punctuate' and not extended. Even if this is so, and it is a debatable point, such sense-data can be *located* by a co-ordinate system (see 3.18) and *bear spatial relations* to other sense-data and this, as will be seen, is what must be established for the purposes of my argument. *Many* sense-data are certainly extended and any *n* such 'punctuate' sense-data ($n > 1$) will form a spatial system, e.g. any three such 'punctuate' sense-data not in a straight line form a triangle. Thus it might be possible to recognise two types of spatial entity: (*a*) extended ones, such as sensory fields, many sense-data and physical objects, and (*b*) unextended ones such as 'punctuate' sense-data which, although themselves un-extended, yet can be *located* by means of a co-ordinate system and bear spatial relations to each other. But, of course, we can also maintain that such 'punctuate' sense-data really are ex-tended, only they are very small. I hold this latter view for the following reason: if a 'punctuate' sense-datum really is not extended—i.e. if it has the geometrical properties of a point—then if we placed a great number of such sense-data close together they could never fuse, for between any two points in a space there are an infinite number of other points. It is, how-ever, an empirical fact that a multiple star is *seen* as a single star; there is only one sense-datum related to the two stars. Further-more in the sense-datum related to a distant nebula the sense-data related to individual stars cannot be made out, and thus they must have fused to form the smudgy homogeneous pale patch which is the sense-datum related to a distant nebula.

2.23. Individual sense-data are, to some extent, arbitrarily chosen parts of the total visual field, which may be taken to be the fundamental unit of structure of this part of the perceptual apparatus.[1] For the visual field may be arbitrarily divided into parts, yet we cannot form a visual field out of any arbitrary collection of separate sense-data. In fact we never come across any sense-data outside a collection of sense-data organised into a visual field, for even hallucinatory sense-data form a unitary field. Imagine, for example, that you are in a totally dark room looking at two adjacent illuminated boards, one painted blue and the other green. Would you describe your sensory experience by saying that you sensed two sense-data—one blue and one green?—or one sense-datum half blue and half green?—or three sense-data, a blue one and a green one surrounded by a black one (so as not to overlook the important black sense-datum related to the dark part of the room)?—or one sense-datum, blue and green in the middle and black round the periphery?—and so on. Clearly the process is one of dividing a given structural whole into arbitrary parts; although some divisions seem more 'natural' than others. This whole field definitely has a shape: it is more or less circular. And it may be divided into sections—i.e. two hemispheres—right and left, or upper and lower; or four quadrants; or into a central region and a peripheral region; etc. Sense-data may be located in any of these regions. Furthermore each sense-datum has a definite position in the visual field during any one specious present: i.e. it may be in the lower right quadrant, or in the upper left quadrant, or partly in one quadrant and partly in another. To say that sense-data are located in determinate positions in the visual field is not a round-about way of saying that physical objects are seen in certain positions in physical space relative to the observer. For these observations are true in the case of hallucinatory sense-data as well as in the case of sense-data related to physical objects. That is to say a visual field filled with hallucinatory sense-data (such as may occur under mescaline with or without the eyes shut) still definitely has a shape and is still divisible into quadrants, and the hallucinatory sense-data still have determinate positions in this field. Hallucinatory sense-data satisfy the axioms of topology just as well as do non-hallucinatory sense-data.

[1] See 8.2 and Chapter 2.

2.24. Sense-data also have shapes and (relative) sizes and may even be subjected to a form of measurement. For instance, we can take as a unit of length the total diameter of the visual field, and we can then observe that every sense-datum will be about $\frac{3}{4}$ or $\frac{1}{2}$ or some fraction of this diameter. Similarly every visual sense-datum may be said to have an area—i.e. such and such a proportion of the total visual field. Thus sense-data can certainly be measured, and these operations conform to Dingle's criterion[1] of what constitutes measurement as any precisely specified operation that yields a number. Measurements of sense-data will never yield any exact number: we cannot say that any sense-datum is an exact fraction of the diameter of the visual field or that it is exactly twice as long as another sense-datum, but then even the most refined physical measurement never yields an exact number.[2] Thus the difference between the measurement of sense-data and the measurement of physical objects lies in the different entities to be measured, the different procedures and rules of procedure adopted to measure them (the measurement of a physical object is constructed from many *alignments* of sense-data), and in the range of numbers obtained by the measurement; they do not differ in any qualitative manner. Measurements of sense-data cannot of course be expressed in inches or centimetres, for these units can only be used in the case of physical objects. Nevertheless the statement 'This sense-datum is more than twice but less than three times as long as that one' may be as true and as certain as any statement made about the relative lengths of physical objects.

2.25. To summarise this list of properties of sense-data: we can say that they are the sort of things (spatial entities) that can bear spatial relations, for they bear spatial relations to other sense-data as well as to after-sensations. Furthermore groups of sense-data are always observed to be organised into wholes—each whole a sensory field—and having relative sizes they can be measured: and, as they *can* be measured, we can argue that (visual and somatic) sense-data *really are* spatial entities.

[1] Herbert Dingle, 'A theory of measurement', *Brit. J. Phil. Sci.*, 1950, **1**, 5-26.
[2] See L. Susan Stebbing, *A Modern Introduction to Logic*, London, 1933, pp. 371-3.

3.   Having given these basic definitions of terms and basic facts about sense-data, we can now proceed to give an account of (3.1) the relation between sense-experience and the physiological processes of perception and (3.2) the relation between sense-data and the brain.

3.1.   Consider a simple experience. You look up at the night sky, look at a star for three seconds and then look away. Concerned in this perception was a series of physical and physiological events including the emission of a series of photons from the star, their long journey to earth and the subsequent complicated events in your retina and nervous system. Also concerned in this perception was an experiential event. The sense-datum related to the star occurred and occupied the centre of your visual field for three seconds and was replaced by another sense-datum when you looked away from the star. The event described by the phrase 'I sensed a sense-datum related to the star' (or 'A sense-datum related to the star occurred in my visual field') thus had a temporal duration of three seconds. Now this experiential event may be divided into a series or class of events. For instance, it may be divided into a beginning, a middle and an end; or into the first second, the second second and the third second; or into the looking that was going on while you were thinking 'that's Sirius' and the looking that was going on while you thought 'no, it's Aldebaran'; or in other ways. So we can ask 'How is the p class of events described in the physical and physiological account of your perception related to the e class of events in your direct experience—that is your experiential events (Def. 6)?' or 'How is the class of events denoted by the phrase "I perceived a star" related to the class of events denoted by the phrase "I sensed a sense-datum related to the star"? How, in general, can a class of events a be related to a class of events b? There are five possible answers.

3.11. a and b may be identical. That is, if any event is a member of a then it is also a member of b and any member of b is also a member of a.

3.12. a can be a proper subset of b. That is, if any event is a member of a it will also be a member of b, but not all members of b are also members of a.

3.13. *b* can be a proper subset of *a*.

3.14. *a* and *b* may intersect. That is they have at least one member in common, and there are members of each that are not members of the other.

3.15. *a* and *b* can be mutually exclusive or disjoint. That is they have no members in common.

3.1. (*cont.*) How then may the class of events *e* be related to the class of events *p*? We can say at once that *e* and *p* cannot be identical, nor can *p* be a proper subset of *e*, for the events of the class *p* have a temporal duration of three hundred years (if we choose a star three hundred light-years distant) whereas the events of the class *e* have a temporal duration of only three seconds. Thus we have shown that the theory of perception known as naïve realism leads directly to a logical fallacy. For it is clearly a logical fallacy to state that a series or class of events with a temporal duration of three hundred years is identical with a series or class of events with a temporal duration of three seconds. Yet the theory of naïve realism states that *e* and *p* are identical. In the case of objects close to the observer this particular argument may be modified as follows: 'Two series of events will not be identical unless the first member of one series has the same time co-ordinate relative to a particular set of co-ordinate axes as the first member of the other series. The first member of any *p* series or class of events (i.e. the physical and physiological events concerned in any particular perception) will always be earlier than (i.e. have a different temporal co-ordinate from) the first member of the *e* class of events concerned in the same perception. Therefore *e* and *p* cannot be identical.' This modification might also be necessary if it is claimed that *e* is identical only with those members of *p* that take place actually on or in the star—i.e. only the emission of photons for a period of three seconds, and not their subsequent journey to earth, nor the subsequent events in the retina and nervous system. This claim, however, is refuted by the second leg of my argument given above. This theory must therefore be discarded.[ab] Thus either (3.16) *e* must be a proper subset of *p* or (3.17) *e* and *p* must overlap or (3.18) *e* and *p* have no members in common. To consider these in turn:

3.16.⁰ To say that *e* is a proper subset of *p* means that some physiological events are experiential events. This is the theory of psycho-neural identity which has been largely abandoned by neurologists (see Brain[1] and Sperry[2]) for the following reason. Two groups of events arranged in a spatial order may not be said to be identical unless they are geometrically congruent. They must be, in fact, but one group of events with two different names or denotations. It has been shown that the events in the cerebral cortex (or in cortico-thalamic projection systems) concerned in a particular perception are geometrically non-congruent with the sense-data that these events are alleged, under this theory, to be. The argument that Brain has used against 'projection' (quoted in 3.1655) can be used to refute with equal finality the theory of psycho-neural identity. The validity of this analysis depends on the truth of the following two statements: (a) *e* is a class of events arranged in a spatio-temporal order, and (b) *p* is a class of events arranged in a spatio-temporal order. Now (a) may be verified by direct observation. The spatio-temporal extension and order of sense-data is sensibly given. There is no reason to suppose that physical events do not possess a spatio-temporal order, although it is not possible to prove this logically (see 4.31). We can either claim that the spatial order of physical events can be verified by indirect observation (for the exact meaning of 'indirect observation' see 4.22) or, if for any reason this is objected to, we can use statement (b) as a fundamental axiom in our system.

3.161. We have thus shown that any particular experiential events (Def. 6) cannot be identical with any physical events. For, as we demonstrated above, they cannot be identical with the physical events (either inside or outside the physical organism) concerned in that perception; and they clearly cannot be identical with any of those physical events—*p'*—*not* concerned in that perception. Let us say that P is the class of all physical events (P = *p* + *p'*). These arguments apply to the patterns of neuronal impulses in the cortex of the older neurophysiology and also to the more highly organised moving patterns involved

[1] Brain, loc. cit. (*a*).

[2] R. W. Sperry, 'The mind-brain problem', *American Scientist*, 1952, **40**, 291–312.

in the scanning processes postulated by McCulloch and Grey Walter. Neurons can be said to form bivalent systems (because it is alleged that they have only two functionally important states—discharge and rest), and their states can be expressed mathematically by means of Boolean algebra. In the cybernetic theories brain function is treated essentially algebraically. Observed complexities of behaviour are attributed to the fact that for n elements there are $2(n^2 - n)$ modes of existence; and the brain consists of some 10,000 million elements. However, there are not only problems of behaviour; there are also problems of experience—particularly of perception. Patterns of neuronal excitation form also *geometrical* figures, and it is these figures that must be correlated in neurophysiology's own theory of perception with the geometrical figures (sense-data) that form the elements of experience. The algebraic formulations of cybernetics have nothing to say on the geometrical problems of relating experiential events to brain events.

3.162. Could we say that the cortex 'learns' in some way that neuronal impulses coming up the optic radiations to the cortex, when the eyes are directed at a circular object, have come from a circular object, although the actual cortical patterns concerned are not circular? Hebb[1] and Pitts and McCulloch[2] have both suggested methods how the brain could, if taught, develop certain invariant responses to certain classes of objects—how it could 'recognise' all triangles, all red objects, etc.—by setting up certain complex circuits in its nerve nets. It is at any rate clear that a good deal of learning has to take place before adult perceptions occur—the experiences of the congenitally blind restored to sight by operation show us this—but can *any* such theory be used to account for the obvious incongruity in spatial structure between sense-data (Def. 1) and their correlated brain events, or rather between one particular sense-datum and its correlated brain event, or between the visual field taken as a whole and the known visual regions of the brain? I do not think so for the following reason. We do not merely gain information about physical objects; there are also sense-data to be observed

[1] D. O. Hebb, loc. cit.

[2] Walter Pitts and W. S. McCulloch, 'How we know universals', *Bull. Math. Biophys.*, 1947, **9,** 127–47.

in the visual field in direct experience whose geometrical and topological properties it is unreasonable to doubt. No arguments based on experience can be used to deny that experiential events do have the properties that they may be observed to have (some of which were listed in 2.2).[d] Any such learning can only be effected by creating new cortical patterns of neuronal excitation (or by creating the potentiality of such new patterns by synaptic changes), which new patterns by themselves, or added to the previous patterns in any possible way, still do not possess a circular spatial structure or anything like one. It should be emphasised that the brain can only do basically one thing and that is to form extremely complex and ever-changing spatio-temporal patterns of neuronal impulses and fluctuating potentials.

3.163. It might be argued (somewhat along the lines of Berkeley's new theory of vision) that we feel the real shape of objects with our hands and the cortex then uses this information to 'interpret' visual stimuli. But we cannot abandon naïve realism in the visual process only to smuggle it back in again when considering somatic sensation. If I trace out a circle with my hand there is nothing circular about the cortical patterns set up by this movement. So the problem is merely transposed to the somatic field for my sensed hand also undeniably describes a circular movement. The brain, in fact, as a machine simply cannot construct the sense-data that, as we have seen, play their part in every perception.

3.164. The fact that the theory of psychoneural identity is wholly untenable has been obscured in the past for the following reasons: Most people interested in the theory have been concerned with problems of mind-brain relation rather than with theories of perception. They have either (3.1641) followed Descartes in holding that a mind is composed of an Ego and its thoughts, or (3.1642) they have accepted a behaviourist analysis of 'mind'. In the former case the problem of relating a mind and a brain appears as the Cartesian dilemma of how may an unextended entity (or 'spiritual substance') be related to and interact with an extended mechanical system such as the physical brain. These same people usually take a naïvely realistic attitude (usually taken over quite uncritically from 'common sense') towards their own sense-data. But even if we accept the Cartesian analysis of mind, we cannot accept the theory of psycho-neural identity, for unextended events not arranged in a spatial order cannot logically be identical with any group of spatial events arranged in a spatial order. If we accept a behaviourist analysis of 'mind', the theory of psycho-neural identity loses all meaning, for there cannot be any psychical events, in a behaviourist analysis, to relate to physical events. But we cannot accept a behaviourist analysis of 'mind', for it is reasonably certain that there are sense-data and that our evidence for the existence of physical objects is based on sensing sense-data. For sense-data play a part in all perceptions, including the behaviourist's perception of his experimental animals.[a] However, as I shall argue below, minds may be held to incorporate sense-data, and the problems of mind-brain relation may best be formulated in terms of the relation of spatial sense-data to the spatial brain. The problem becomes one of relating two sets of extended entities.

3.165. Another factor that has obscured the fact that the theory of psycho-neural identity is whólly untenable has been the invention of the concept of the 'projection of sensations'. Ruch has described this as follows:[1]

'All of our sensations are aroused directly in the brain, but in no case are we conscious of this. On the contrary, our sensations are projected either to the exterior of the body or to some peripheral organ in the body, i.e., to the place where experience has taught us that the acting stimulus arises. The exteroceptive sensations are therefore projected exterior to our body. Sound seems to come from the bell, light from the lamp, etc. . . . An important aspect of sensation which deserves to be called the *law of projection* is that stimulation of a sensory system at any point central to the sense organ gives rise to a sensation which is projected to the periphery and not to the point of stimulation.'

Since the final result of this process is evidently a spatial and organised entity (sensum or percept) it would seem a necessary condition for the validity of this theory that some spatial process

---

[1] T. C. Ruch, in J. F. Fulton's *Textbook of Physiology*, 16th ed., Philadelphia, 1950, p. 311.

of the organism would effect this most complex process of projection. It is notorious that nothing like this has ever been detected. In fact, as Brain has argued,[1] it is very hard to believe that such a process actually occurs. The chief objections that can be laid against the postulate that there is such a process of 'projection of sensation' are as follows:

3.1651. It appears to have no basis in physics. No physical entity is projected and the projection itself is not a physical process. For, if Ruch's 'sensation' (which is alleged to be projected) is a physiological entity or process it should be constructed of neuronal impulses (in however complex combinations) or some activity (or even inactivity) of nerve cells and fibres. Neither nerve cells nor fibres, neuronal impulses, atoms, molecules, radiation, nor any chemical, electrical or physical activity of any kind is projected from the cerebral cortex into the external world, except some minute electrical fields which no one has ever suggested mediate the alleged 'projection' of sensations. What else is there to project? No one has ever detected or measured this process in the laboratory. Since it is not a physiological process at all what possible status could it have?

3.1652. Ruch's introduction of the concept of learning to account for the phenomenon implies that in the child sensa are actually in the brain, but at some time during development they leave it and get projected into external space. This merely postpones the development of this process that has never been empirically detected. Now it might be admitted that nothing is really projected in a literal sense, but that the concept of projection of sensations is a metaphorical way of saying that the brain 'knows' that physical objects seen are spatially external to its own physical organism. We are here using 'know' in the sense of having gleaned a basic operational rule or item of information from its past working, just as a computing machine might abstract such an item of information not specifically fed to it (we do not *teach* children that physical objects are exterior to their bodies) from the total complex of information fed into it during its working life. But this would not explain the basic fact that 'projection' requires the first and the last members of

---

[1] Brain, loc. cit. (*a*).

a causal chain to be identical events, which is logically impossible. As Russell says:[1]

'Whoever accepts the causal theory of perception is compelled to conclude that percepts are in our heads, for they come at the end of a causal chain of physical events leading, spatially, from the object to the brain of the percipient. We cannot suppose that, at the end of this process, the last effect suddenly jumps back to the starting-point like a stretched rope when it snaps.'

3.1653. It may be argued that it is superfluous to postulate a process of 'projection of sensations' since a proper attention to the internal detail of the physiological theory itself eliminates the necessity for making it. The somatic sensory field,[2] which is merely the collection of all somatic sensa (touch, pain, pressure, thermal; skin, muscle, bone, joint and visceral sensa) that is sensed during any specious present, is unreflectingly identified by 'projection' theorists with the physical organism. As visual sense-data (sensations) are clearly topologically outside the somatic sensory field, if the latter is taken to be the physical organism, then processes must be invented whereby the visual sense-data somehow get to be outside the physical organism. If, however, we identify both visual and somatic sense-data with events in the brain or with events in the mind, there will not be any need to talk about the projection of anything. For, if sense-data are in the brain, the fact that visual sense-data are topologically external to somatic sense-data need only be explained by pointing out that the visual parts of the brain (in which visual sense-data are held by this theory to be located) are topologically external to the somatic sensory parts of the brain (in which this theory likewise locates somatic sense-data). And if sense-data are in the mind, the fact that visual sense-data are topologically external to somatic sense-data is merely a basic fact about the mind not standing in need of any explanation (see also 3.32).

3.1654. If we ask for the *evidence* for the projection of sensations,

---

[1] Bertrand Russell (*c*), *The Analysis of Matter*, London, 1927, p. 320.
[2] The somatic sensory field is often called the 'body image' in neurology: see Chapter 3.

a reply might be given thus: 'It is known that if any sensory nerve is stimulated (say the ulnar nerve at the elbow) the sensation is not felt at the site of stimulation, but it is felt in the field of distribution of that nerve, e.g. in the hand and not in the elbow. This is a matter of common knowledge. Similarly tumours in the temporal lobe may give rise to hallucinatory sounds heard outside the head; lesions in the occipital lobe may give rise to hallucinatory sights seen outside the head; etc.' The assumption made here, of course, is that normal sensations, such as a touch on the little finger, and the sensation felt on stimulating a sensory nerve, such as a blow on the 'funny bone', are both *located* in the *physical* hand. But if we deny this assumption, the need to postulate the projection of sensations disappears. We can see now that the concept of 'projection' has arisen out of a muddled attempt to combine the physiological account of perception with the 'common sense' account. This is done by extending the causal chain of perception by yet another step; that of projecting the sensation back into the external world. This leaves the status of the sensation completely mysterious; for it cannot be identical with the external physical event (that which is seen) concerned in the perception, for the first and last members of a causal chain cannot be identical events; and it cannot be identical with the brain events concerned in the perception, for the sensation has specifically been projected from the brain. The only cure for this kind of muddle is to develop a logically coherent and empirically valid neurological theory of perception without incorporating, in an uncritical way, any of the miscellany of folk beliefs and popular superstitions about how the perceptual apparatus functions that constitute, to so great an extent, the 'common sense' account of perception.

3.1655. Brain's argument is as follows:[1]

'Thus when we perceive a two-dimensional circle we do so by means of an activity in the brain which is halved, reduplicated, transposed, inverted, distorted, and three-dimensional. If physiological idealism is to be really physiological it must admit that its theory of projection breaks down because the

---

[1] Brain, loc. cit., p. 9.

circle which is said to be projected from the cerebral cortex never existed there at all.'

So we can conclude that there is no such process as the 'projection' of sensations at all.

3.17. If e and p intersect then those members of p that are e must clearly be brain events (for the reasons given against 3.11 above). Therefore some members of e must be brain events. But there is surely no possible phenomenological classification of experiential events into those that are brain events and those that are not. Furthermore, we saw in (3.16) that no members of e can be identical with those members of p that are·brain events. Therefore e and p cannot intersect.

3.18. Thus by elimination we have established the statements 'e and p have no members in common' and 'e and P have no members in common'.[1] How, then, are we to relate e and p? We noted above that all members of e are spatial entities[2] which bear spatial relations to each other and e may be described as a *spatial system*. A spatial system may be defined as a group of spatial entities that bear some specified spatial relation R to each other. In the case of visual sense-data this relation—R1—will be given below. Physical objects are also spatial entities and form a single spatial system where R is the following relation:— All physical objects can be so related to a system of co-ordinate axes OX, OY, OZ set at right angles to each other anywhere in the physical universe that they can be located uniquely in terms of a co-ordinate system obtained by using these axes (this will be relation R2). If we include time we can use four co-ordinate axes; OX, OY, OZ, and OT. (See also the footnote to 3.182.) Now it is clear that if e and p have no members in common then their members must form different spatial systems. For if e and p are mutually exclusive classes, then R1 and R2 will be mutually exclusive relations. That is to say no sense-datum can be located by using the set of co-ordinate axes OX, OY, OZ (for *any* value of the temporal co-ordinate). Yet sense-data

[1] In these arguments we are not including those members of p beyond the reach of the most powerful telescopes, for clearly they could not be members of e in any case.

[2] All members of e are experiential events and any experiential event is a change of state of a sense-datum which is strictly the spatial entity.

can certainly be located by using a set of co-ordinates. The visual field of contiguous sense-data may be divided into quadrants (right upper, right lower, left upper, left lower), and sense-data may be located in one or other part of one or other of these quadrants. This quadrantic division of the visual field is in everyday use in neurology and is used to indicate the position of hemianopias, quadrantic field defects, etc. A more elaborate system may be constructed as follows. Two mutually perpendicular straight lines may be traced on the glass of one lens of a pair of spectacles. The sense-data related to these lines, when the spectacles are placed before the eyes, will form co-ordinate axes for the visual field and can be made to intersect at the foveal point (provided that the eye is not moved in the orbit). Arbitary numbered intervals can be marked on these axes, and a grid formed by perpendiculars drawn through each numbered interval on each axis may be marked on the glass. Using the sense-data related to this grid any sense-datum can be located in the visual field by indicating the co-ordinates of the points on the grid that it occupies. These numbers can never be exact, but then no location of a real physical object can ever be absolutely exact (in contrast to the 'location' of an imaginary point), for there are unavoidable 'experimental errors' in any physical measurement. The location of sense-data is only quantitatively different and not qualitatively different from the location of physical objects, which we saw was also true in the case of measurements of sense-data and physical objects (see 2.24). Thus we can give the relation (R1) to define the spatial system of sense-data: 'Sense-data are so related to the co-ordinate axes of the subjective visual field that they may be located in terms of a co-ordinate system obtained by using these axes.' These co-ordinates have been termed the co-ordinates of the subjective visual field by Bender and Teuber.[1] How then are we to relate the OX, OY, OZ co-ordinate axes of physics, *for any particular value or values of the temporal co-ordinate* (the preceding 10 words will be represented by the symbol ϕ below), to the co-ordinate axes of a (subjective)

[1] M. B. Bender and H. L. Teuber, 'Spatial organisation of visual perception following injury to the brain', *Arch. Neurol. Psychiat.*, 1947, **58**, 721–39.

visual field? In other words what are the spatial relations between these two sets of spatial axes at *any* time-instant? As these axes define different spatial systems this can only be done in two ways:

(3.181) There may be no spatial relations between the two sets of axes.

(3.182) The two sets may be conjoined to determine a single six-dimensional manifold.

To consider these in more detail:

3.181. We must allow a different set of co-ordinate axes for the visual field belonging to each individual; for my sense-data are not contiguous with your sense-data. If, then, we wish to locate all the events in the universe to include experiential events as well as physical events, we must use $(m + 1)$ sets of co-ordinate axes in the case of m human individuals (with three spatial [and one temporal axis] in each set[1]). The total Universe of events would then consist of the physical world (composed of stars, planets, trees, physical human bodies including brains, etc.) and, for m individuals, m experiential worlds (each composed of sense-data and images, thoughts, affects, $\pm$ a Pure Ego). All these worlds would be quite separate and their contents would be held to bear no spatial relations to each other but only temporal relations, causal relations and relations of class membership.

3.182. Alternatively it may be the case that each private experiential world is not spatially isolated from the others and from the physical world, but that the contents of each world (world $\equiv$ spatial system) are spatially related and the various spatial systems form, for m human individuals, a single $(3m + 3)$ dimensional spatial manifold (or a $4m + 4$ dimensional spatio-temporal manifold if we include time). Thus to give an account of all the spatial relations in the Universe we need a system of $(3m + 3)$ co-ordinate axes. If we wish to locate all the entities in the Universe, we can start by erecting one set of axes OX,

---

[1] If an additional axis (or axes) is (or are) used to represent time, then all these different spatial systems may share a common time axis or each may have a different time axis. But the discussion of this point is beyond the scope of this book.

OY, OZ (ϕ) to locate all physical objects. Then we can erect another set of three axes (ϕ) each of which is at right angles to each of OX, OY, OZ to locate the sense-data and images of one human individual.[1] Then we can erect a third set of axes (ϕ) each of which is at right angles to each of the six preceding axes to locate the sense-data and images of a second human individual. This process is merely continued until we have come to the last of the finite class of human individuals. To say that a spatial system is x-dimensional is to assert that x co-ordinates are necessary to locate the position of any one point (or object or entity) in the system. In our case a more convenient way of doing this would be to use the co-ordinate system of physics as at present to locate objects in the physical world. Then if we wanted to locate a sense-datum or an image belonging to a particular human individual A in relation to his other sense-data, we would use three other co-ordinates having erected three new axes (ϕ). The O point for this new set could be placed anywhere in the spatial system of his visual or somatic sense-data or amongst his images. We would then have merely to define the relation between these two sets of axes (as in 3.181 or 3.182). Then if we wished to locate a sense-datum in B's visual field in relation to the sense-data in A's sensory fields and in relation to the objects in the physical world, we would erect a further set of three axes (ϕ) with an O point anywhere among B's sense-data or images. We could then express the location of any of B's sense-data and images in relation to the rest of his sense-data and images by reference to these axes, and we could express their location in relation to A's sense-data and images and in relation to physical objects by defining the relations between B's set of axes and A's set and the set used for locating physical objects in the physical world: and similarly for the individuals C, D, E, etc. The co-ordinates of the total $(3m + 3)$ dimensional system (ϕ) would then be collected uniquely into sets of three (ϕ), and the location of objects in it would not need the cumbrous system of $(3m + 3)$ co-ordinates (ϕ), but this could be

[1] Values of ϕ here will be limited by the dates of the birth and death of the individual—unless any sense-data and images of any pre-natal or post-mortem state of that individual's mind continue to bear spatial relations to physical objects.

done by indicating which set of axes we were proposing to use (A's, or B's, or C's etc.), and by defining the relation between this set of axes, those belonging to the other individuals B, C, D, etc. and between all these and those that we use to locate objects in the physical world.

In either case we are dealing with a far-reaching development in cosmology. For each statement asserts (in more 'common-sense' language) that there is not one Space-Time (as is thought at present) but that there are many Space-Times. In (3.181) the physical universe becomes but one of many spatial universes in which events ordered in a spatio-temporal system occur. In (3.182) the physical universe becomes merely a section of the total spatio-temporal Universe of events. Thus, to give a proper account of experiential events and their relation to brain events, we may have to exchange the four-dimensional geometry in current use in cosmology for an n-dimensional geometry.

3.2.   The relationship between sense-data and physical objects may be analysed in a comparable way. It was noticed above that sense-data may be observed by any one individual during any one specious present to be spatial entities arranged in a spatial system and to bear spatial relations to other sense-data. Physical objects may also be assumed to be spatial entities arranged in a spatial system and they bear spatial relations to other physical objects. Now a spatial entity must either (a) bear or (b) not bear a spatial relation to another spatial entity. If (a) holds in the case of sense-data and physical objects, then it follows that (α) sense-data must be identical with external physical objects or at least with parts of them; or (β) sense-data must be identical with parts of the brain; or (γ) they must bear higher-dimensional spatial relations to physical objects. If (b) holds in the case of sense-data and physical objects, then sense-data must be spatially external to the physical world. I have given reasons for rejecting (α) and (β) and so we must accept either (γ) or (b).

3.3.   All this discussion may be summarised in the form of two formal cosmological theories:

I. 'Sense-data and images are spatial entities distinct from physical objects and bear temporal and causal relations but no spatial relations to physical objects.'

II. 'Sense-data and images[1] are spatial entities distinct from physical objects and bear both temporal and causal relations and higher-dimensional spatial relations to physical objects.'

3.31. A more rigorous definition of an n-dimensional system runs as follows:[2]

3.311. 'The empty set has the conventional dimension $-$ 1.;

3.312. The dimension of a space is the least integer n for which every point has arbitrarily small neighbourhoods whose boundaries have dimensions less than n.'

Now, if we consider the spatial systems of the sense-data and images of m individuals and physical objects under Theory I, we can say that, whereas each is three-dimensional (ϕ) ($n = 3$ in 3.312), no point in any of these systems has any neighbourhood in any of the others: thus we are dealing with a collection of separate and distinct three-dimensional spaces or spatial systems (ϕ). In the case of m individuals under Theory II the spatial system composed of all their sense-data and images as well as physical objects is $(3m + 3)$-dimensional (ϕ) ($n = (3m + 3)$ in 3.312), for all points in each spatial system (each of the m private sensible spatial systems + the one public physical spatial system) have neighbourhoods in every other spatial system.

3.32. We can now define what we mean by a mind:

Definition 8. 'A mind is a complex composite of sense-data organised into sense-fields, together with images, thoughts, affects and perhaps a Pure Ego.'

The mind thus defined is a part of the total organism—an extra part which we have previously failed to recognise because of its particular geographical location and because some of its constituent parts (sense-data) have been confused with physical objects. These misidentifications have arisen partly out of our failure to realise that the spatial universe is not necessarily

---

[1] Operationally defined co-ordinate axes as described above are always particular physical entities (such as rays of light) or particular sense-data or images. Thus the spatial relations between these various sets of axes given above are but special instances of the spatial relations of their companion sense-data and physical objects.

[2] K. Menger, *Dimensionstheorie*, Leipzig, 1928, quoted by G. J. Whitrow, 'Why physical space has three dimensions', *Brit. J. Phil. Sci.*, 1955, **6**, 13–31.

limited to the collection of physical objects located in the physical world. There may well be many different three-dimensional spatial (or four-dimensional spatio-temporal) systems of sense-data and images in addition, as described in Theory I. There are also higher-dimensional geometries available to describe the $(4m + 4)$-dimensional spatio-temporal system of Theory II.

3.4. These theories are compatible both with the theory of psycho-neural interaction (in that brain events and experiential events are postulated to be in causal relation) and with the theory of psycho-neural parallelism ('pre-established harmony' could equally well serve to keep the events in each world 'in step'): not that there need be, on a Humean analysis of causation, any essential difference between interaction and parallelism, for all that we really have to deal with in each case is an invariant sequence of events. The traditional theories of interaction and parallelism are theories about the causal relations between psychical events and brain events. Whereas the theories here presented are theories primarily about the *spatial* relations between experiential events and brain events.

3.5. It has previously been suggested on many occasions that sense-data are 'in the brain' or 'in the mind'. For instance, Russell states:[1] 'Whoever accepts the causal theory of perception is compelled to conclude that percepts are in our heads, for they come at the end of a causal chain of physical events leading, spatially, from the object to the brain of the percipient.' Chisholm asks:[2] 'Perhaps we should say that all of them [the sense-data belonging to a table] exist in the mind—or in the brain. But, in this case, what becomes of the table and how can one know anything about it?' and again '. . . the theory of the dualist is that sense-data are "in the mind" or possibly that they are "the brain seen from its metaphysical insides" '. Similarly Russell Brain[3] arguing from the empirical phenomenon of the so-called 'phantom limb' asks: 'What reason, then, have we for thinking that the qualitative and spatial characteristics of sense-data related to a limb which is really there are not similarly

[1] Lord Russell, loc. cit. (*c*), p. 320.

[2] Roderick M. Chisholm, 'The theory of appearing', in *Philosophical Analysis*, Max Black, ed., Ithaca, 1950, pp. 104 and 112.

[3] Brain, loc. cit. (*a*), pp. 12 and 7.

generated elsewhere; for example, in the brain or the mind of the observer?' 'The facts of neurophysiology are held to mean that sense-data are "really" located either in the cerebral cortex or in the mind of the observer.' However, the meaning of these statements 'sense-data are in the brain' and 'sense-data are in the mind' has never been made very clear, nor have their implications been properly developed. We can interpret the statement 'sense-data are in the brain' as stating the theory of psychoneural identity, which holds that spatial sense-data are spatial parts of the brain. We have reviewed the reasons that have been given for rejecting this theory. The statement 'sense-data are in the mind' is of no great novelty but it tends to lead those people who accept it as being true into idealism. However, this theory has suffered from the following crippling difficulty. The mind in the traditional Cartesian theory is both non-spatial and un-extended—extension being the cardinal attribute of physical things. If a mind, ontologically distinct from the physical body, is a non-spatial entity ('thinking substance'), then, if sense-data are to be 'in the mind', they must also be non-spatial. Yet the spatiality of sense-data is given no less than their colour. If the mind is thought to be non-spatial how can spatial sense-data and images belong to such a mind? How can that which is spatial belong to that which is non-spatial? How can an entity be both wholly non-spatial and spatial and how can a non-spatial whole be composed of spatial parts? This real dilemma has remained hidden by a pseudo-dilemma 'How can the unextended and non-spatial mind and the extended brain interact?' Ducasse has argued[1] that this is not a dilemma at all for the reason that no *a priori* statements about causal relations between events (or between entities of any kind) are justified and these relations may only be determined by empirical methods. There is no *a priori* reason why a non-spatial entity should not react with a spatial one. But there is also no *a priori* reason why the mind, if it is ontologically distinct from the brain, should be a non-spatial entity.

Ayer deals with the suggestion that 'sense-data are in the mind' in the following manner. He asks,[2] 'But what is meant

[1] C. J. Ducasse, *Nature, Mind and Death*, La Salle, 1951.
[2] A. J. Ayer, loc. cit., p. 76.

here by saying that an object exists in the mind? Presumably that it is what we should ordinarily call a state of mind.' And again,[1] 'How indeed the mind is supposed to contain them [the objects of which we are sensibly aware], it is not easy to understand. I do not think that even Berkeley can really have wished to maintain that "sensible qualities" were literally inherent in the mind as in a region of space.' We can see how this dilemma has arisen. People commonly suppose that their sense-data belong to the external world around them and that their minds are composed solely of their thoughts, attitudes, feelings, etc., which do not seem to be extended. Then, if they ask themselves 'How can my sense-data be in my mind?', they think of this question in terms of this other question 'How can my sense-data be some sort of thought or feeling—how can they be *states* of mind?' But this is the wrong way to approach the whole problem. To say that sense-data are in the mind is to suggest that the mind consists not only of thoughts and feelings but of sense-data as well. It is futile to attempt to reduce sense-data to states of thoughts or feelings. For sense-data and images are spatially extended and feelings and thoughts are not.

4.   OBJECTIONS TO THESE THEORIES[*]

4.1.   A contemporary philosopher might ask 'Why is it necessary to introduce the complications of the sense-datum terminology? In common speech all perceptual experiences can adequately be described by using ordinary words like ⟨see⟩, ⟨look⟩, ⟨hear⟩, etc. The meaning of these common-sense words is set and established by their correct usage in English and it is impossible to deny that these words have these meanings. Furthermore the objects of our perceptions are physical objects—ordinary material things such as tables and chairs—and nothing so recondite as sense-data.' This is perfectly correct but it is unsatisfactory for at least three reasons:

4.11.   If we make this analysis of perception we may be able to describe all our sense-experiences in a manner intelligible to other people, but we will not be able to give any logically coherent account of how the physical and physiological processes

---

[1] Ayer, loc. cit., p. 77.

31

concerned in perception are related to my visual experience. For to attempt to do so along these lines leads us into the logical fallacy discussed in (3.1).

4.12. It is true that as long as one uses common-sense terms like ⟨see⟩, ⟨look⟩, ⟨hear⟩, etc., it may lead to confusion if one uses them in any way that is not governed by correct English usage. Unfortunately, however, in actual English usage, the words ⟨see⟩, ⟨look⟩, ⟨hear⟩, etc. are used to describe hallucinatory sense-experiences as well as veridical ones. I am not referring here to people whose wits are bemused by drink or delirium who, it might be claimed, were no longer in a state to observe properly or to adhere to correct English usage. I am referring to the extensive factual evidence available in the reports of those experimental subjects who have taken mescaline. These subjects can of course distinguish between their hallucinations and their veridical perceptions but that is not the point. Philosophers who claim that it is only correct to say that we see physical objects (we must say that we 'have' hallucinations or some such) have not studied what people who are having hallucinations under such experimental conditions actually say. The only criterion for correct usage in English is to find out what most people in the circumstances under consideration in fact say. Since people describing their hallucinations almost invariably say 'I see' and not 'I seem to see' or 'I have', it is as much correct English usage to say 'I saw a flower' when the flower was hallucinated as when it was a botanical flower. A study of what people say when they have hallucinatory experiences of the type called *apparitions* yields the same results; e.g. 'I saw him as clearly as I am seeing you now.' Therefore *seeing* cannot simply be taken as a perceptual relation between people and physical objects; for it is not the case that, in all instances of *seeing*, it is physical objects that are seen.

4.13. Thirdly, now that we have a definition of ⟨sense-datum⟩ we can surely ask that *some* account be offered of the relationship between sense-data and physical objects.

4.2. An important objection to all forms of the causal theory of perception has been made by Ayer.[1] He states that his analysis

---

[1] Ayer, loc. cit., pp. 220–1.

has shown that causal relations must always be relations between events

'which are capable, at least in principle, of being observed. To attempt to make use of causal laws in order to infer from the occurrence of observed events to the existence of things that are outside the scope of any possible observation is not merely to put forward hypotheses for which there could not be any valid evidence; it is to extend the use of the concept of causality beyond the field of its significant application. And it is this that constitutes the fatal objection to all forms of "the causal theory of perception"; for it is characteristic of all the theories that are commonly brought under this heading that the causes of what is actually observed are assumed themselves to be, in principle, unobservable.'

Ayer says that this fallacy is involved in the case where the external cause is thought to be an unobservable 'physical object' as well as in the cases where it is thought to be God. However, as against this we can argue as follows:

4.21. The neurologist need not use causal laws to infer that physical objects are ontologically distinct from sense-data. He can do this by showing that the spatio-temporal structure of any e is different in any particular case from the physical events it is related to, i.e. to all the members of p that are concerned in that perception. Thus e cannot be identical with these physical events and thus one must be in some sense exterior to the other. No causal *laws* as such are involved.

4.22. Ayer's argument may be interpreted as stating that the causal theory postulates the existence of events or things which it is logically impossible to observe, and that this entails a logical contradiction. For it is held that a thing which it is logically impossible to observe is nothing. However, the causal theory can distinguish between *direct observation* and *indirect observation*. We can say that 'directly to observe an object or event' is synonymous with 'to sense a sense-datum (or examine an image)', and that 'indirectly to observe an entity or event' is synonymous with 'to perceive a material thing'. The causal theory of perception does not then require us to say that physical objects are *unobservable* things-in-themselves. It has only to postulate that physical objects are ontologically distinct from sense-data (are things-in-themselves), and that the relations between sense-data and physical objects are such that, by sensing some sense-data (not hallucinations), we perceive material things and so gain knowledge about the physical world. The nature of these relations has been further discussed elsewhere (in 3 and 7). The particular reasons why we cannot observe physical objects directly are given in (7), and the particular change in the conditions of our perception that would enable us to do this is described in Appendix I.

4.3. We must also deal with two other objections that have been made against the causal theory of perception. These run as follows: 'If all that you can observe directly are sense-data how do you know that there are any other entities such as physical objects if you can never observe these directly? If you accept the causal theory then you cannot escape solipsism.' And 'How do you know that sense-data are different from physical objects if you can never compare them directly?'

These objections can be answered in the following manner:

4.31. If I say 'Physical objects are external in some sense to my sense-data' then I cannot prove deductively from this premiss, and from what I can observe from a study of my sense-data, the existence of a physical world external to these sense-data; but neither can I disprove it. In order to substantiate the charge that this analysis of perception leads *inevitably* to solipsism, it would be necessary to show that it could be proven that there could not logically be any entities or events external to my sense-data.[1] This cannot be done for, as Hume showed, one cannot logically prove or disprove the existence of things. Any enumeration that I can make of all the existent entities in my solipsistic universe will constitute a finite series—I can only count the finite number of sense-data that form my experiential events—and I have no logical guarantee that this list will include all the existent entities that there are. The mere fact that I can say 'There is a series of events $a^1 - a^2 - a^3 \ldots a^n$ which includes all my experiential events does not logically entail that there are *no*

---

[1] It is evident that no empirical investigation could demonstrate that there could not logically be any events external to my sense-data.

other series of events $b^1 - b^2 - b^3 \ldots b^n, c^1 - c^2 - c^3 \ldots$
c^n, etc. I can give a logically coherent account of my experience
by supposing that the universe consists only of the most complex system of sense-data, images, thoughts and feelings that
form my experiential events. The extremely complex order of
these *need* not be explained by reference to any 'world' external
to this collection. It would merely be the case that these sense-
data, images, thoughts and feelings happen to be arranged in
this particular way. Furthermore, the order of these events *need*
not be explained by any reference to physical objects made up
by, or in causal relation with, these sense-data. For the order
inherent in the whole system of sense-data, images, feelings and
thoughts would be such that certain visual sense-data merely
happen to be associated with certain other visual sense-data,
with certain auditory sense-data, with certain images, affects
(feelings), etc.; certain thoughts would merely happen to be
associated, at various times, with various sense-data, affects,
etc.; certain affects with certain combinations of sense-data and
thoughts; etc., etc. But the fact that the order of my experience
does not logically *need* to be accounted for by reference to any
'external world' does not logically entail that it would be a
logical fallacy to account for it in this way. For, as was argued
above, the solipsist has no valid grounds whatever for holding
that there *cannot be* any events or entities external to his own
sense-data, images, feelings and thoughts. Such other entities
or events could therefore bear causal relations to his sense-data
or could themselves be other sense-data associated with other
people, just as his own sense-data are associated with himself.
Thus all that I can do is to inspect my own sense-data and say
'It is logically possible that these are the sum total of reality.
It is also logically possible that there are entities and events
exterior to these sense-data and causally related to them. I am
perfectly free to adopt whichever I consider gives me the best
explanation of the world.'

4.311. One suppressed argument underlying the charge that
the causal theory of perception as I have presented it leads inevitably to solipsism is as follows. If I examine my private
sense-data and say 'This is the universe—there are no entities

or events outside these', then there cannot be any such events outside these sense-data, because I have taken up all the space there is to contain these sense-data, and there is none left over for any other entities or events;[1] and, as it is thought that there cannot be any non-spatial entities or events, it seems to follow that there cannot be any other entities besides my sense-data, because there can be only one three-dimensional spatial system in the world. However, this presupposition is unjustified as we have seen (3).

4.312. Furthermore we might be asked, 'How do you know that a physical object related to a certain round sense-datum is itself round and not, e.g., square?' In order to be pertinent this questioner would have to propose that, owing to some specific process in the perceptual mechanisms, *every* square object is represented by a round sense-datum. For, if it was the case that only a few people's round sense-data represented square objects, and all other round sense-data represented round physical objects, then we could explain these eccentric instances by saying that they were merely curious perceptual anomalies due to defects in the perceptual mechanisms. That is to say, mechanisms could evolve which transformed round patterns of excitation at the retina into square sense-data in the part of the human representative mechanism which corresponds functionally to the screen of the television set: but these aberrant mechanisms could be regarded as freaks. Similarly, if it were claimed that the perceptual mechanisms were so unstable that they sometimes represented round, and at other times square, physical objects by round sense-data, then we should be able to observe some of our round sense-data changing into square ones and vice-versa —which we do not. It would clearly be implausible to claim that the representative mechanisms of perception arbitrarily represented some square physical objects always by square sense-data and others always by round sense-data and never confused these; and, moreover, the same selection, as to which square physical objects were to be represented by square sense-data and which by round ones, would have to be made by the

[1] An example of this argument may be found in Berkeley, *Principles*, 67. Note further that the solipsistic universe is still a spatial universe.

perceptual mechanisms belonging to everybody; otherwise we would frequently disagree as to the real shapes of physical objects—which we do not in this degree. So our questioner must say that all square objects are represented by round sense-data. In this case we would soon find out the true state of affairs by scientific means. For instance, if a string is tied to a stone and the stone is whirled round, we would sense a square sense-datum related to the path of the moving stone, whereas the laws of motion would indicate that this path *must* be *circular* and not *square*. It can be argued that if everyone saw round physical objects, or the circular paths of moving physical objects, as squares, that nevertheless the correct laws of motion for the physical world would have been reached in time. For instance, the elliptical planetary orbits, whose form is relevant to the laws of motion, were never perceived as wholes but were plotted from frequent observations of the positions of small points of light; and thus the particular sensory transformation we are concerned with here would not have been relevant. Similar arguments can be constructed to show how similar constant sensory transformations in the case of the other primary qualities of objects might have been discovered by scientific means. In the case of the secondary qualities of objects the problem does not arise; for physical objects are not to be thought of as literally coloured or 'sounding' or smelly. Thus we can claim that, in the case of the primary qualities, our guarantee that physical objects do correspond to the sense-data which represent them, is that their mathematical properties discovered by observation and experiment do correspond, within certain limits, to the mathematical properties of the sense-data. In the case of the secondary qualities, the physical correlate is wholly to be sought in terms of certain physical properties of the objects (absorption of light, emission of volatile oils, etc.) which take part in the causal chains of perception. It is clear that something of this kind has been taking place in the discovery of the constant size effects, the anisotropy of visual space, etc. (see Chapter 2).

4.32. It is in any case sterile to demand that, in science, the truth of our basic assumptions be logically certain. We must be satisfied with a reasonable degree of certainty. In the construction of the scientific world scheme we do not select a number of logically certain statements from which to start, but we construct an interlocking series of statements (descriptions of observations, various level hypotheses, laws, etc.), the truth of any one of which is not logically certain, but each of which is reasonably certain and which form a coherent whole, the reasonable certainty of each part of which supports the reasonable certainty of the other parts. We are dealing, in other words, with empirical statements and not with the analytical statements of logic and mathematics. Thus it is no very pertinent criticism of a scientific theory of perception to point out that one of its basic assumptions is not logically certain but only reasonably certain. It is a much more serious criticism of a rival theory to point out that it contains a statement that we are all reasonably certain is false—i.e. that we are immediately aware of the surfaces of external physical objects or with the objects themselves. This statement is incompatible with another statement the truth of which is reasonably certain—i.e. that the velocity of light is finite.

4.33. The sceptical question asked at the beginning of 4.3 can be rephrased as follows: 'What can be the relation in a particular perception between a sense-datum and a physical object whereby the sense-datum can give us veridical non-inferential information about the physical object?' This question can be put in more general terms: 'How can we obtain information about one set of events *f* by observing another set of events *g* in such a way that we could be said to be directly observing *g* and indirectly observing *f*?' In the physical world we find that this can be done by the use of special mechanisms which we can call *non-symbolical representative mechanisms*.[1] In these the information is transmitted by the construction by the mechanism of black-and-white or coloured patterns which reproduce the shapes, relative sizes, spatial relations and shades or colours of the objects at the input of the mechanism. We do, in fact, gain a quantity of knowledge about objects and events by means of the representative mechanisms of the cinema and television without ever having seen

[1] To be distinguished from symbolical representative mechanisms such as the telegraph.

these objects and events directly[1] and without ever doubting the validity of this knowledge. I know, for instance, what Mr. Gary Cooper and Mr. Alec Guinness look like as well as I know what my grocer and my butcher look like, although I have seen the latter face to face but never the former. Therefore we may make a considerable advance towards solving the problem of perception by showing that the physiological mechanisms concerned in perception *are* non-symbolical representative mechanisms.

It is thus possible to illustrate the distinction that I have drawn between the direct observation entailed in sensing sense-data and the indirect observation entailed in perceiving material things by using the analogy of television. Imagine that you are in a darkened room watching the screen of a television set on which a programme is being presented. You could describe your experiences in either of two ways. You could say, 'I am watching a number of lines glowing on a curved opalescent screen. These lines are continually changing their intensity of illumination and the shadows and highlights thus produced are making patterns that I can recognise represent people moving about in a room.' Or you could say, 'This afternoon I saw Arsenal playing Manchester United and now I am watching a fashion show'; or 'I am now getting a much better view of the coronation procession than I would have got if I had joined the crowds lining the route.'

Thus watching a televised event can be analysed in terms of seeing a series of lines of light of variable intensity of illumination glowing on an opalescent screen or of seeing the actual events televised. I will now suggest that sense-data may bear the same kind of relation to physical objects as the 'images' on a television screen bear to the actual people and scenery in the studio. We can postulate that the causal processes concerned in perception work in a manner similar to the manner in which television works. As Grey Walter says:[2] 'In other words, the televisual system behaves very much like the neuro-visual one.'

---

[1] ⟨seeing directly⟩ is equivalent to ⟨observing indirectly⟩ in the technical sense of the latter given in 4.22.

[2] W. Grey Walter in *Perspectives in Neuropsychiatry*, D. Richter (ed.), London, 1950, p. 77.

The following objections may be raised against this analysis of perception:

4.331. It may be claimed that the statement that vision works like television does not avoid the epistemological problem. For, it will be argued that, whereas we can always verify that the 'images' on the television do, in fact, represent what is going on in the television studio merely by going to the studio and seeing for ourselves directly, we can never confirm by direct observation any such postulated relation between sense-data and physical objects lying external to them. No one, it can truthfully be said, has ever observed, either directly or indirectly, a sense-datum in any kind of spatial relation with the physical object that it represents. But it is only empirically impossible to do this and not logically impossible as will be shown in Appendix I.

4.332. It might be said that we only recognise the 'images' on the television screen because we have on some previous occasion seen the real objects directly. However, we do not have to have seen the physical object directly in order to be able to recognise it: it is enough to have seen a picture or other representation of the object. For instance, it would be a simple matter to recognise a giraffe from its picture without ever having previously seen a giraffe. This entails, however, that someone must have seen the giraffe in order to photograph it or paint it. But suppose an animal which no one had ever seen before were photographed by a trip-wire camera. Would we not then say that veridical information had been obtained by means of a representative mechanism of an object which no one had ever seen (directly)? Similarly it can be argued that we only accept television pictures as veridical representations of some physical events on the unconscious or barely conscious premises that we know the general principles of the mechanism concerned and that, if we care to, we can always go to the studio and confirm what is going on there by 'seeing for ourselves': and we cannot do this in the case of vision. However, consider the following case. Suppose that we take a child at birth and encase its head in a device so that opposite its eyes covering what will subsequently be its whole field of vision is the screen of a television set. The television camera would be located on the farther side (relative to the face of the child) of the screen opposite the eyes (it will be helpful to imagine that owing to technological advances we can make the operative parts of the mechanism very small and light). Then there is no reason to suppose that the child would not be able to lead a fairly adequate visual life. It could see anything in range of its television camera, and it would gain all manner of knowledge about the world by visual means, in spite of the fact that it would have had no 'direct' experience[1] of any physical object except the screen of the television set before its eyes on which the representation of external events is cast by the proper mechanism. It would react to its visual stimuli like any other child before it knew anything about the nature of its predicament or how television worked. Clearly its knowledge of the world and its reactions to it would not in any sense depend on its knowledge about the nature of the mechanism presenting all its visual experience. If we were subsequently to tell the child about the actual state of affairs, this would not invalidate any of its previous knowledge of the world obtained by vision. Thus it is logically possible to gain knowledge about external physical objects without ever having seen any of these objects directly and without realising that we have never seen one directly (for we would take care to bring the child up without letting it realise that it was different to other children by taking such precautions as always wearing similar masks ourselves in her presence, etc.).

4.333. It may further be said that the analogy of television is 'only an analogy'. To this we can reply that the statement 'the causal physiological processes of perception work in a manner similar to television' is a statement of the kind 'the heart works like a pump' or 'the arms work like levers' and not of the kind 'he worked like a beaver' or 'I felt like a worm'. That is to say this analogy is not a poetical or metaphorical way of saying something which it would be misleading to take literally. The statement 'the heart works like a pump' means 'the heart is a pump' which means 'there are mechanisms which we call pumps according to the mechanical principles underlying their

---

[1] Adopting, for the moment, the naïve realist terminology.

construction and to what they do. Some of these are artefacts, like village pumps, and some are found in living organisms, like hearts.' Similarly we can say, 'There are mechanisms that we call television mechanisms. Some of these are artefacts, like commercial television sets and some are found in living organisms such as parts of the central nervous system.': and we are now in a position to 'test the analogy' by presenting empirical evidence that suggests the mechanisms of visual perception *are* television mechanisms (this will be done in 10.2).

4.334. It might be said that the 'television' theory of perception applies only to inner details of cerebral mechanics, and that it would not be inconsistent to hold both that these cerebral mechanisms do function in the manner described by neuro-physiologists and that in our every-day perception we do ob-serve physical objects directly. But it does not seem very plaus-ible to assert that, whereas physiological processes are necessary conditions for our perception of external physical objects, our perception of such objects is nevertheless a process in some manner different from the physiological processes and can employ principles that would be incompatible with those used in the physiological account. For if the perceptual apparatus func-tions according to the principles used also in television, or any other representative mechanism, then it cannot also function wholly as a simple optical instrument, which it must do if it is to give us a direct view of physical objects. For it is both logic-ally and mechanically impossible for a television mechanism to provide a direct view of the objects and events televised. The lens of the eye and related parts are, it is true, simple optical devices, but these form only a small part of the perceptual apparatus. The rest of the perceptual apparatus cannot function both as a representative system and as a simple optical device.

To this the naïve realist might reply that his account of per-ception does not at all require that the central nervous system should be an optical instrument, but only that, in Hirst's words,[1] '. . . the events of the causal chain cause a person to see a book or some such object, . . .', and again:[2]

[1] R. J. Hirst, 'Perception, science and common sense', *Mind*, 1951, **60**, p. 494.

[2] Hirst, loc. cit., p. 503.

'... we may say that perceiving is a relation between person and external object such that a complex of brain activity is caused in him by the object, and he has a complex experience which is to be considered the same event as the brain activity, and which seems to the person concerned to be awareness of the external object and some of its characteristics. Somewhat similar brain activity and so somewhat similar experiencing may occur without an external object as cause, as in dreams, eidetic imagery and hallucinations.'

But, as we saw in (3.16), considerations of neuroanatomy forbid us to identify the complex spatial entities that are veridical and hallucinatory percepts with the spatial patterns of neuronal impulses in the brain concerned in these perceptions. If it is claimed that perception is a non-spatial act—that the brain processes merely are the act of perception divorced from its spatial content of physical objects, hallucinations, dream 'images', etc. —the puzzle remains of how can the *spatial* patterns of neuronal excitation be identical with any such *non-spatial* act of perception. Furthermore, Hirst does not explain how 'the person concerned' is related to his own brain activity. If we interpret 'person' to be a synonym for 'total organism' or 'whole brain', there is no reason why certain patterns of neuronal activity in the brain should seem to the organism, or to the brain, to be parts of external objects, or an awareness of external objects; or even what it means to talk of the 'awareness' of an organism or brain, or of 'seeming' in connection with an organism or a brain in this sense. And if 'person' does not mean 'total organism' or 'whole brain', it cannot mean anything in this context, unless we suppose it to denote a Cartesian mind, in which case there it is even less intelligible to say that certain neuronal patterns in the brain seem, to the Cartesian mind, to be an external physical object or an awareness of an external physical object (see also 10.223).

4.4. I stated above that it was my aim to show that all theories other than those presented here seeking to relate experiential events to the physiological causal chain of perception led to logical fallacies. However there is one account of perception that avoids this difficulty: we can abolish all experiential events. We can say that there are causal chains of physical events leading from external physical objects and from organs inside the body to the brain. In the brain the patterns of nervous impulses coming from the sensory receptors that form part of this causal chain are integrated and analysed by the computing mechanism of the brain. This mechanism has two outputs: one via the motor cortex to the muscles, so that appropriate (learned) responses can be made to the pattern of sensory input; and one via the motor speech area, so that appropriate statements can be made: and we can claim that nothing else whatever goes on.[1] There are no perceptions, sense-data, images, phenomenological objects, sensations or thoughts if any of these are postulated to be anything or any process other than the physical and physiological events of the causal chains of perception in the physical world. If, for example, a subject reports that he is observing a certain kind of after-sensation, all that is happening is that a certain pattern of activity reverberates in his visual cortex and this pattern translated to the motor speech centres give rise to articulated responses similar to those that would have been given had such a cortical pattern been set up by an input coming from a certain pattern of coloured lights. All alleged experience can be treated in a similar manner. Now it must be noted that this account only succeeds by abolishing all experience. For the objects that purely naïve view of perception takes to be actual physical objects cannot under this theory exist at all. When I open my eyes I seem to be confronted with a variegated field in which a number of 'objects' simply are located. Yet under this theory none of this gay panorama has any existence. It is not even hallucinatory. Such 'objects' could only be *past* states of physical objects and physical objects do not exist in the past. All the 'objects' apparently presented directly to me when I open my eyes are already in the Limbo of the past. The real physical objects are in the *future* relative to every one of these 'objects'. These 'objects' are not even illusory or hallucinatory or imaginary. There is just nothing whatever there at all. 'But', it may be claimed, 'surely I can notice a difference between what I experience when I open my eyes which seems to one to be a variegated field of objects and the darkness when I close my

[1] The emotional mechanisms can be considered as providing complicated ways of influencing the motor mechanisms.

eyes?' This presents no difficulty to this theory. For with the eyes open certain patterns of neural stimulation (schemata) translated from the visual cortex to the speech centres lead to statements such as 'I can see a variegated field of objects' and when the eyes are shut the quite different schemata that arise in the visual cortex lead to different statements such as 'it now seems all black to me' when translated to the speech centres.[1] Thus when someone (A) opens his eyes and says 'I can see all these physical objects directly' and I say 'There is nothing there; what is really there is *future* to all the objects that you think you are seeing directly': in our two cases different response patterns are aroused in the speech centres in response to similar patterns in the visual centres. It is not difficult to describe mechanisms whereby the brain can distinguish true from false statements (on a basis of logical fallacy or unattained predictions etc.) by making an analysis of its own schemata. My response is compatible with the known facts about the time that perceptual processes need to take place and A's response is not.

It may be further claimed (i) that we can be certain that there are experiential events and that phenomenological objects do exist for it may be claimed that it is indubitable that in sensory experience we are confronted with something and not nothing or (ii) we could be said to be cutting off the branch on which we sit for it will be said that all our knowledge about brains, etc. is obtained by sensory experience and thus such knowledge cannot be used to deny that we do have such experience. However, we can reply to (ii) by saying that our knowledge depends on receiving physical excitation of sensory receptors from objects and not on having 'experiences', for our knowledge consists of nothing more than what the organism can write or say in response to various stimuli. Now if objection (i) is to be maintained the claimant must give some account, in a logically coherent manner, of what it is he claims to experience and of the relations between his experiences and the physiological processes of perception. My argument in this chapter is that there are only two ways of doing this as expressed in Theories I and II.

[1] The schemata responsible for these utterances occurring in the brain without producing actual motor excitations may be considered to be thought.

It is also logically consistent to deny the existence of any experiential events, for it can always be claimed that the apparent certainty we feel about the existence of experiential events is only the occurrence of certain patterns in the symbolising centres of our brains and these patterns are 'false' in the sense described above. It is only mistaken to try and make the best of both worlds by claiming that experiential events could be identical with brain events or that brain events are identical with something mysterious called a 'perception' of a physical event, etc. The choice between the radical behaviourist theory and the theories evolved here can only be made by experiment—possibly along the lines suggested in Appendix I. It may be noted that solipsism is also logically tenable and deals with the problem in a manner opposite to the radical behaviourist theory, i.e. by abolishing all physical events.*

5.   Various authors have suggested that perceptual space ('private space', 'the space of sense-data', etc.) is a different space to physical space. However, these statements have not been based on, and have not led to, a thorough analysis of what it means to say that one 'space' is different from another 'space' and how exactly perceptual 'space' is different from 'physical' space. It is, in any case, a mistake to attempt to relate the 'space' of sense-data to the 'space' of physical objects, for that is to hypostatise space. We can only talk about spatial entities that do or do not bear spatial relations to each other and that may form spatial systems defined by some spatial relation R (see 3.18).

5.1.   A theory similar to Theory I has been used by Price[1] to relate images and physical events. He says 'Mental images, including dream images, are in a space of their own. They do have spatial properties. Visual images, for instance, have extension and shape, and they have spatial relations to one another. But they have no spatial relation to objects in the physical world.' This theory about the spatial relations between images and physical objects can be shown to have as a necessary consequence my Theory I for a continuous spatio-temporal transformation series can be traced between visual sense-data and

[1] H. H. Price (*a*), 'Survival and the idea of "another world" ', *Proc. Soc. Psychical Research*, 1953, **50**, 1–25.

images. For visual sense-data are spatio-temporally continuous with their after-sensations. Under mescal I have observed (directly) an after-sensation turn directly into a typical mescal hallucination or sensory image. I was looking at the grates of my gas fire in London which was of the modern type and had a grid composed of small squares glowing brightly in the flame. When I shut my eyes the after-sensation was a grid formed of little pale squares and these changed as I watched into a pyramidal pile of glass spheres, each sphere of perfect form and bearing one prominent highlight. Mescal images are a highly developed form of hypnagogic images which, in turn, merge imperceptibly into ordinary visual images.[1] So we must agree with Schilder when he says:[2] 'Thus eidetic images like other images, lie in the same space as percepts. The space in which objects are perceived, and the space in which they are imaged, are one and the same.'

Price does not however suggest that images can bear higher-dimensional spatial relations to physical objects.[3]

'If I dream of a tiger, my tiger-image has extension and shape. The dark stripes have spatial relations to the yellow parts, and to each other; the nose has a spatial relation to the tail. Again, the tiger image as a whole may have spatial relations to another image in my dream, for example to an image resembling a palm tree. But suppose we have to ask how far it is from the foot of my bed, whether it is three inches long, or longer, or shorter; is it not obvious that these questions are absurd ones? We cannot answer them, not because we lack the necessary information or find it impracticable to make the necessary measurements, but because the questions themselves have no meaning. In the space of the physical world these images are nowhere at all. But in relation to other images of mine, each of them is somewhere. Each of them is extended, and its parts are in spatial relations to one another. There is no *a priori* reason why all extended entities must be in physical space.'

The fallacy contained in this argument is the supposition that

[1] J. R. Smythies, 'The "base-line" of schizophrenia', *Amer. J. Psychiat.*, 1953, **110**, 200–4.
[2] Paul Schilder (*a*), *Medical Psychology*, New York, 1953, p. 41.
[3] Price, loc. cit. (*a*), pp. 11–12.

all spatial relations must be expressible in metrical terms or in terms of comparative length; i.e. that *a* is three inches from *b* or that *a* is longer or shorter than *b*. There are, however, topological relations such as *inside* and *outside* which are not expressed in these terms. All points in a cube transected by a plane not in the plane are outside the plane. Any line connecting any of these points on the same side of the plane will also lie outside the plane. Such a line will bear spatial relations to any line in the plane, although this relation might seem mysterious to any Flatlanders[1] living in the plane. Similarly there is no *a priori* reason why there should not be higher-dimensional spatial relations between sense-data and images on the one hand and physical objects on the other.

5.2.   Broad has formulated Theory II as follows:[2]

'The difficulty which we feel about the ontological status of sensa may be put as follows: We feel that anything which can successfully claim to be "real", must be some*where* and some*when*. And we are so much accustomed to physical Space-Time, and to the way in which physical events and objects occupy regions in it, that we think that an event cannot be "real" unless it occupies some region of physical Space-Time in the way in which a physical event does so. Now, it seems clear that either (1) sensible determinates (such as some particular shade of red) do not inhere in regions of physical Space-Time, but in regions of some other Space-Time; or (2) that, if they do inhere in regions of physical Space-Time, they must inhere in the latter in some different way from that in which physical determinates (like physical motion) do so. Either there is one sense of "inherence" and many different Space-Times, or there is one Space-Time and many different senses of "inherence". On either alternative the world as a whole is less simple than we should like to believe; and, if we have come to think that there is only one possible Space-Time and only one possible kind of inherence, we shall be inclined to suppose that sensa are nowhere and nowhen, and therefore are mere fictions. Since this is plainly contrary to fact, unless the whole way of treating sensible appearance which is developed in this book be wrong, we must accept one of the two alternatives mentioned.'

---

[1] See E. A. Abbott, *Flatland. A Romance of Many Dimensions*, Oxford, 1926.   [2] C. D. Broad, loc. cit (*b*), pp. 543–4.

And again:[1]

'For reasons already stated, it is impossible that sensa should literally occupy places in scientific space, though it may not, of course, be impossible to construct a space-like whole of more than three dimensions, in which sensa of all kinds, and scientific objects, literally have places. If so, I suppose that Scientific Space would be one kind of section of such a quasi-space, and e.g., a visual field would be another kind of section of the same quasi-space.'

However, it is not necessary to call a space of more than three dimensions 'space-like' or a 'quasi-space'; it is merely an '*n*'-dimensional space where $n > 3$. In this *n*-dimensional space Scientific Space and a visual field would not be two different *kinds* of section but would merely be two different sections. If we decide to talk about the spatial relations between spatial entities instead of 'spaces' we see that Broad's first alternative is equivalent to Theory II.

5.3.   Russell refers in a number of places to the fact that perceptual space is different from physical space. For instance in *Human Knowledge* he says:[2]

'An even more serious error, committed not only by common sense but by many philosophers, consists in supposing that the space in which perceptual experiences are located can be identified with the inferred space of physics, which is inhabited mainly by things which cannot be perceived. The coloured surface that I see when I look at a table has a spatial position in the space of my visual field; it exists only where eyes and nerve and brain exist to cause the energy of photons to undergo certain transformations. (The "where" in this sentence is a "where" in physical space.) The table as a physical object, consisting of electrons, positrons, and neutrons, lies outside my experience, and if there is a space which contains both it and my perceptual space, then in that space the physical table must be wholly external to my perceptual space. This conclusion is inevitable if we accept the view as to the physical causation of sensations

[1] Broad, loc. cit. (*b*), pp. 392–3.
[2] Bertrand Russell (*d*), *Human Knowledge, Its Scope and Limits*, London, 1948, pp. 236, 238 and 241.

A.P.—E   49

which is forced on us by physiology and which we considered in an earlier chapter. . . .'

'All this, I say, has long been a commonplace, but it has a consequence that has not been adequately recognised, namely that the space in which the physical table is located must also be different from the space that we know by experience. . . .'

'The objects of perception which I take to be "external" to me, such as coloured surfaces that I see, are only "external" in my private space, which ceases to exist when I die—indeed my private visual space ceases to exist whenever I am in the dark or shut my eyes.'

This last quotation contains an important fallacy. When I shut my eyes my private 'space' does not cease to exist. The complex and varied visual field that I notice when my eyes are open is merely replaced by a reddish spatial datum, which fills the whole field, and inside which spatial after-images of the brighter objects, that I was looking at when my eyes were open, fade away. When I go into a dark room my visual field is filled with a single very dark sense-datum in which I can frequently detect faint clouds of colour floating about and sometimes little hypnagogic images. Galton has put this clearly:[1]

'I should have emphatically declared that my field of view in the dark was essentially of a uniform black, subject to an occasional light-purple cloudiness and other small variations. Now, however, . . . I have found out that this is by no means the case, but that a kaleidoscopic change of patterns and forms is continually going on,' . . .

Furthermore in both these situations my somatic sense-data are still with me and these are certainly spatial.

5.31. In *The Problems of Philosophy* Russell says that sense-data are situated in our private spaces. He continues:[2] 'Thus we may assume that there is a physical space in which physical objects have spatial relations corresponding to those which the corresponding sense-data have in our private spaces. It is this physical space which is dealt with in geometry and assumed in physics and astronomy.' But it is a mistake to suppose that geometry

---

[1] Francis Galton, *Enquiries into Human Faculty*, London, 1883, p. 158.
[2] Russell, loc. cit. (*b*), p. 49.

refers only to physical 'space'. Geometrical statements about sense-data can certainly be true or false and not meaningless.[1] Many of the statements of geometry refer in any case to unrealised 'pure' circles and other figures. The ratio of the circumference to the diameter of any circular physical object will never be π and neither will this ratio hold for the relation between the circumference and the diameter of any circular sense-datum. But certain topological propositions do hold for physical objects as well as for sense-data.

5.32. In *Mysticism and Logic*[2] Russell introduces the idea of a six-dimensional space. He states that the space of one man's sensible objects and the space of another man's sensible objects are different spaces and not merely different parts of the same space. He goes on to suggest that there are a multitude of three-dimensional spaces in the world and 'although these spaces do not have to one another the same kind of spatial relations as obtain between parts of one of them, it is nevertheless possible to arrange these spaces themselves in a three-dimensional order'. He then goes on to describe how the whole world of particulars is arranged in a six-dimensional space[3] 'that is to say, six co-ordinates will be required to assign completely the position of any given particular, namely, three to assign its position in its own space and three more to assign the position of its space among the other spaces'. I do not think that Russell really means to suggest in this argument that my sense-data bear higher-dimensional spatial relations to physical objects or to your sense-data. It is possible to argue that these statements of Russell's are meaningless since he uses ⟨space⟩ as a noun and talks about spatial relations between 'spaces'. He seems to be using the word ⟨space⟩ to denote the system of spatial relations between spatial entities, and to say that objects are in different spaces would then mean that the spatial relations between these entities (physical objects), as perceived by one man, are not the same as the spatial relations between the same objects, as perceived by another man at the same time. If, however, we

---

[1] Jean Nicod (loc. cit.) bases geometry on the spatial relations discernible between sense-data.

[2] Bertrand Russell (*e*), *Mysticism and Logic*, London, 1918.

[3] Russell, loc. cit. (*e*), p. 139.

re-phrase Russell's statements in terms of spatial entities bearing spatial relations to other spatial entities, an ambiguity is at once disclosed. For he says that it does not appear probable that two men[1]

'ever both perceive at the same time any one sensible object'; and that it follows from this that 'the space of one man's objects and the space of another man's objects have no place in common, that they are in fact different spaces, and not merely different parts of one space. I mean by this that such immediate spatial relations as are perceived to hold between the different parts of the sensible space perceived by one man, do not hold between parts of sensible spaces perceived by different men. There are therefore a multitude of three-dimensional spaces in the world: . . .'

Now it can be seen that there are two different questions here that Russell has failed to disentangle. These are (5.321) 'Are the spatial relations between sense-data in my visual field exactly the same as the spatial relations between sense-data in your visual field when we are standing close together and looking at the same scene?' The answer to this will clearly be 'no' but this fact does not give us any reason to postulate any six-dimensional spaces to explain why things appear to have different shapes or different spatial relations to other things when viewed from different places. (5.322) The second question runs as follows: 'Do my sense-data bear any "ordinary" spatial relations to your sense-data?' By this I mean 'Does any one of my sense-data bear the same sort of spatial relation to any one of your sense-data that this sense-datum of mine bears to other sense-data of mine, that your sense-data bear to each other and that physical objects bear to each other?' If we answer 'yes' to this question then there is still no need to talk about 'private spaces' or 'six-dimensional spaces' or 'a space of perspectives', etc. For we can say that sense-data merely are, or are parts of, physical objects, and the physical objects that I see certainly bear spatial relations to the physical objects that you see. But if we answer 'no' to this question then it seems that we are committed to either Theory I or Theory II. For we are suggesting that the

[1] Russell, loc. cit. (*e*), pp. 138–9.

proper way to say 'my private space is a different space to your private space' is to say 'none of my sense-data bear any spatial relations to your sense-data'; or it is to say 'My sense-data bear higher-dimensional (i.e. not "ordinary") spatial relations to your sense-data', and thus 'the spatial system composed of my sense-data and images during one specious present and the spatial system composed of your sense-data and images during the same specious present form a six-dimensional manifold (ϕ).' If we talk about a six-dimensional 'space' we must mean a spatial system which is the sixth in the series of which the line, plane, volume and hypervolume form the first four members. It must be a system of six-dimensional solids or at least a collection of objects of less than six dimensions arranged in a six-dimensional spatial order.

The 'all-embracing' three-dimensional space of physics cannot be a logical construction (as Russell suggests) out of a crude space of six-dimensions.[9] For it is the crude space of six dimensions (ϕ) that is all embracing (so long as only one individual is involved), since it contains all physical objects and all the sense-data and images of that individual as well. In the case of m individuals only a $(3m + 3)$-dimensional space can be all embracing. In Russell's six-dimensional universe it is assumed that the private sensible spaces of m individuals form a single three-dimensional manifold. But surely each individual has a different sensible space from those of other individuals, for my sense-data are not contiguous with those of other people.

5.4. Moore makes a most interesting remark in *Philosophical Studies* the implications of which however he does not pursue.[1]

'. . . for it seems to me just possible that the two sensibles in question [that belonging to a florin and that belonging to half-a-crown], though *not* circular *in my private space*, may yet be circular in *physical* space; and similarly that though the sensible of the half-crown is smaller than that of the florin *in my private space*, it may be larger *in physical space*.'

But he goes on from here to enquire into the meanings of the word ⟨see⟩ rather than to enquire how one space can be different from another space and in particular how his private space

---

[1] G. E. Moore, *Philosophical Studies*, New York, 1922, p. 187.

(and my private space and your private space) differ from physical space and from each other.

5.5. Similarly, Ayer[1] makes a brief reference to the fact that both John Stuart Mill and Berkeley fail 'to distinguish properly between physical and sensible space' but he does not analyse this proposition further.

6. AN ELEMENTARY DEVELOPMENT OF PSYCHOPHYSICAL GEOMETRY

Take any point A in the visual field of an individual and take any point B in the physical world.

6.1. Then if the theory of naïve realism is true the following propositions are true:

6.11. A can be the same point as B; that is A and B can be different designations of the same point.

6.12. There will always be at least one line in the physical world parallel to the line AB joining A to B (when $A \neq B$).

6.13. Take any other point C in the physical world. Then the angle ABC may be any angle between 0 and 180° (when $A \neq B$).

6.2. If the theory of psycho-neural identity is true the same set of propositions are true.

6.3. If Theory II is true then the following set of propositions are true:

6.31. A cannot be the same point as B.

6.32. There will be no line in the physical world parallel to AB.

6.33. The angle ABC will always be a right angle.

6.4. If Theory I is true then this third set of propositions will be true:

6.41. A cannot be the same point as B.

6.42. There can be no line joining A to B.

6.43. There can be no such angle as ABC.

6.5. The point A can be taken as the infinitesimal limit of dPs

[1] Ayer, loc. cit., p. 246.

in Fig. 1 and the point B can be taken to be the infinitesimal limit of dPh in the same figure (see Appendix II).

7.   It will be necessary to outline something of the possible nature of the causal process postulated by both these theories to connect sense-data and images to the brain. I will adopt Thouless and Wiesner's[1] terminology to this end. The symbol ψ will denote *the causal processes that connect the brain with the spatial system that is the mind.*[2] The symbol ψ_y will denote *the processes that connect the sensory areas of the brain to the sense-fields of direct experience.* Subsections of ψ_y similarly connect the brain to images, feelings and thoughts. The symbol ψ_x will denote *the process whereby the 'will' is transmitted to the motor cortex and 'voluntary' movements are initiated.*

7.1.   I will consider Theory I first. This holds that there are no spatial relations between sense-data and images on the one hand and physical objects on the other. The processes of causal connection between brain and mind thus become *non-spatial causal processes* crossing the unimaginable void between the public physical spatial system and each private experiential spatial system. This void is literally unimaginable, for we naturally cannot comprehend it by means of our spatial imagination. We can only understand that such a void is possible on a purely conceptual basis. We can understand that the Universe may be composed of a great number of three-dimensional spatial systems (or four-dimensional spatio-temporal systems) none of which bear any spatial relations to any of the others.

7.2.   If, on the other hand, Theory II describes the actual state of affairs then the nature of the ψ processes become more complicated. For we must distinguish between two possible alternative forms of the theory.

7.21.   Theory II A. The spatial system of sense-data and images (of one individual) is finite. That is to say there can only be a limited number of distinguishable sense-data in the visual field and somatic sensory field of one individual during one specious

---

[1] R. H. Thouless and B. P. Wiesner, 'The PSI-process in normal and "paranormal" psychology', *Proc. Soc. Psychical Research*, 1947, **48**, 177–96.

[2] The symbol ψ does not stand for the description 'the causal processes etc.' It stands for these processes themselves.

present. Yet any spatial system is potentially infinite in spatial extent, or, if not infinite, it can be much larger than the very limited sensible extension of the sensory fields. Thus it is quite possible that sense-data and images are surrounded topologically by unsensed entities which form an unsensed spatial system, just as a small bubble of air can be surrounded by, or embedded in, a large amount of water. Each private *sensed* spatial system may thus be set in or embedded in a larger unsensed system of the same dimensionality (i.e. the same set of three spatial axes may be used to locate uniquely any point in the unsensed system as is used to locate any point uniquely in the sensed system). We can call this larger system the *psychical spatial system*. Part of its contents (i.e. some of the entities that make up the whole collection of spatial entities which bear spatial relations to each other and form the psychical spatial system) may then be supposed to form the unsensed part of the non-symbolic representative mechanism which builds up the visual field in the manner suggested by the stroboscopic patterns (see 10.2) and which builds up the other sensory fields. The sensed part of this mechanism *is* the visual field of contiguous sense-data and the physical part is the sensory nervous system. The unsensed part of this mechanism would then bear much the same kind of relation to the sensed part as the 'works' of the television set bears to the images on the television screen and the screen itself. Such unsensed psychical entities would remain unsensed because they would geographically be so located and structurally so related to the visual field that they would be hidden by it.

That which can be sensed must be located spatially in a sensory field which is the last stage of the perceptual apparatus. That which can be perceived must be materially present to the external sense-organs—that is, it must be a member of the physical spatial system. 'Psychical mechanisms' could not therefore be sensed, because they would not lie spatially in the visual field but would lie spatially outside it (or behind, or beyond it), and they could not be perceived, because they would not be members of the physical spatial system and could not be materially present to the external sense-organs (the barrier that prevents us from perceiving them is the same that prevents a Flatlander from 'seeing' events in the cube surrounding the plane that are not in his plane). But such 'psychical mechanisms' could nevertheless be structural parts of the perceptual apparatus, linking the brain to the sensory fields.

Such unsensed psychical entities would also bear higher-dimensional spatial relations to physical objects, and their spatial system would be separated from the spatial system of the physical world by a dimensional interface. Any two three-dimensional (or n-dimensional) spatial systems which together make up a more than three-dimensional (or $(n + x)$-dimensional) system will have a dimensional interface between them. A simple example is provided by a cube intersected by a plane. The surface of the plane directed toward the cube is the dimensional interface. If we imagine two-dimensional beings living in the plane—the inhabitants of Flatland—their universe will be bounded not only by the edges of their plane but also by the surface that the plane presents toward the cube and which forms the dimensional interface. This would be quite apparent to us but the Flatlanders would be quite unaware of its existence. Similarly our physical universe may be separated from each of our private universes by a dimensional interface, and our own private universes may be separated from those of other people by other dimensional interfaces.[1] Such dimensional interfaces represent limits set on the movement of objects and entities by the limits of their extension. Thus physical objects could not enter any psychical world, nor could sense-data enter the physical world, but an n-dimensional being could move any entity into any other space system. Normally the only transdimensional processes are conducted by ψ_y and ψ_x which correlate the phenomena occurring in all these worlds. There is no problem about how such processes could react with the brain as every point in the brain can be contiguous with the unsensed psychical mechanism. Thus we can summarise this discussion by saying that ψ_y and ψ_x may be wholly spatial causal processes connecting the brain to the sensory fields.

7.22. Theory II B. Sense-data and images might still bear higher dimensional spatial relations to physical objects, yet

---

[1] A universe may be defined as a three-dimensional spatial system (or a four-dimensional spatio-temporal system). The Universe may be defined as the totality of all universes.

there would not be any such unsensed psychical spatial system as postulated in Theory II A. ψ would then be a non-spatial causal process as described in Theory I. The sense-data and images of each individual would form a self-contained, limited and finite universe spatially outside the physical universe. That is to say that the Universe would still be a $(3m + 3)$ dimensional spatial system (ϕ) (as it is in Theory II A) and not a collection of entirely separate three-dimensional universes (ϕ) (as it is in Theory I). But each private universe would be limited only to what can be sensed (as it is in Theory I). Under Theories I and II B there is no unsensed psychical spatial system.[1] The only difficulty here is the fact that the non-symbolical representative mechanisms of perception would contain a non-spatial part connecting two spatial parts: the brain and the sensory fields. There is no *a priori* reason, however, why this should not be the case, and these theories are perhaps to be preferred on the principle of Occam's razor. But these various theories may lead to different predictions, only one of which can be confirmed by experiment, and then we will be able to choose between them on empirical grounds. Until then we can only indicate what is possible. (See Appendix I.)[h]

8. The theories presented here have the following advantages over the traditional Cartesian dualism:

8.1. The Cartesian theory can give no intelligible account of the relation that sense-data bear to the brain nor the role that they play in perception. It can be argued that Descartes made the mistake of confusing a part of the mind (the Ego and its thoughts) with the whole mind.

8.2. In these new theories mind and body can still be considered to form a single and unitary organism of which they are different spatial parts, thus keeping to the neurological dictum that each human individual is a single organism. The sensory fields of contiguous sense-data are certainly organised and are postulated by these theories to be structural parts of the perceptual

[1] Theory I can also be divided into a Theory I A and Theory I B with respect to the existence or non-existence of unsensed psychical entities as was Theory II, in which case what I have called Theory I above is really Theory I B.

apparatus, for they form the final terms in the spatio-temporal causal processes of perception.

8.3. The Cartesian dualism is a dualism of substance whereas the theories presented here are dualisms of spatial location. They are however monistic theories in the logical field of causal relation and organisation. They make no mention of the mediaeval concept of substance.

8.4. It should be possible to investigate the causal relations between a brain and a mind by constructing an 'n'-dimensional physics based on an 'n'-dimensional geometry, just as current physics is based on a 4-dimensional geometry. The general problem is how may one group of spatio-temporal events affect another group of spatio-temporal events when the members of one group either bear no spatial relations or higher-dimensional spatial relations to members of the other group? If the requisite physics can be constructed, then it may be possible to make predictions based on these theories that can be tested by experiment.

9.   SUMMARY AND CONCLUSIONS OF CHAPTER I

These theories have been constructed by a combined logical and empirical analysis of perception. We have shown that sense-data (Def. 1) cannot, for sound logical reasons hinging on the empirical fact that the velocity of light is finite, be identical with the external physical objects that they represent: nor can they, for equally sound logical reasons hinging on the anatomy of the brain, be identical with any parts of the brain. If we introduce a temporal factor we can state that experiential events (Def. 6) cannot be identical with any physical events for the same reasons. Yet sense-data are spatial entities that bear spatial relations to other sense-data. We are therefore forced to abandon the assumption that we can locate every event in the universe by using one set of four co-ordinate axes. We must use, for m human individuals, either one set of $(4m + 4)$ co-ordinate axes or $(m + 1)$ sets of four co-ordinate axes to locate all experiential events as well as all physical events in their correct mutual spatio-temporal relationships. Furthermore, if we postulate that minds are ontologically distinct from brains, we are not forced to say that minds must be non-spatial entities ('ghosts in machines'). It is true that the Ego and thoughts do not appear to be extended, but they may only form a part of each individual mind. For spatial sense-data and spatial images may also be parts of each individual mind. We can thus suggest that an individual mind may consist of a spatial part (sense-data and images) in intimate association with a non-spatial part (thoughts, affects and perhaps a Pure Ego). Each living human being would then be composed of a physical body, a member of the class of physical objects, and a mind, the two related by relations of class-membership, causal and temporal relations and perhaps spatial relations.

An alternative theory of radical behaviourism is also developed. This is logically tenable and capable of fitting the facts. But the abolition of all experiential events is a desperate expedient and is liable to meet with the same kind of 'blank incredulity' as is invoked by Mill's theory of matter as the permanent possibility of sensations. A theory which does not have to go to such extremes may perhaps be preferable on this account alone, but it may be possible to confirm the theories presented here by experiment.

Thus it may be that an accurate and comprehensive neurological account of perception cannot be given solely in terms of physical objects including brains and the language system of physics, but it may have to include ⟨sense-datum⟩ among its basic terms. In Woodger's analysis[1] it cannot use only the physical-object language, but it must include the sensible-object language as well. The rules for combining these two languages may be based on the postulated relations between physical and sensible objects outlined above. Furthermore we have no need to use vague and undefined terms to describe the final phases in the afferent causal chain of perception. We do not have to say that cerebral events cause a 'sensation' (or 'impression', 'conscious experience', Lockean 'idea', 'image', etc.) to arise in the mind (or in 'consciousness', 'in direct awareness', etc.). Nor do we have to postulate that cerebral events 'underlie' mental events, or form a mysterious 'substratum' for them. We can say

[1] J. H. Woodger, *Biology and Language*, Cambridge, 1952.

that particular cerebral events concerned in a particular perception cause particular sense-data to occur in a visual field. We can give an outline of the further spatial relations that may relate sense-data to the brain. Neurology is surely concerned with the actual functions of the brain which may be better understood if we can establish a particular theory of mind-brain relationship. It cannot merely be assumed that neurology is based on the theory of psycho-neural identity, for neurology itself has refuted this theory.

In the next chapter we will consider the evidence from neurology which shows that the visual field is not merely 'given' as a simple and unanalysable direct view of the physical world, but that it is actively constructed from simpler elements, and that different processes in this construction are linked to different parts of the brain. Most of this evidence may best be accounted for by a representative theory of perception of the kind outlined in this book. Chapter 3 will be concerned with somatic sense-data and their relation to the neurological concept of the body-image.

In the rest of this book the radical behaviourist theory will not be taken into account in order that the alternative theories may be developed fully.

Chapter Two

THE GENESIS OF THE
VISUAL FIELD

10. PHILOSOPHERS, in their analysis of perception, have tended to interest themselves very largely in people with normal brains, and they do not take into their account the many changes in perception that can take place as a result of brain injury and disease. Price[1] brings forward an argument against accepting the evidence from physiology as a basis for any system of knowledge about the nature of perception—'what seeing and touching themselves *are*'. No such system of knowledge, he says, could possibly be more certain than the knowledge obtained from an examination of sense-data themselves. He argues that all physiology is based on the physiologists' sensing of their own sense-data and[1]—'Since the premises of Physiology are among the propositions into whose validity we are enquiring, it is hardly likely that its conclusions will assist us.' This argument cannot be applied, however, to the evidence from neurology, for this deals with abnormal perceptual processes themselves. Thus the neurologist in this field does not deal primarily with facts about the physical world discovered by normal perception but with abnormal sense-data themselves, viz. those sensed by people who have damaged brains. This evidence *is*

[1] H. H. Price (*b*), *Perception*, London, 1950, p. 2.

gained by the normal perception of the neurologist, as when he listens to what his patients tell him or looks at what they draw. Nevertheless the facts discovered (relevant to our enquiry) are primarily *sensed* facts about sense-data and how the complete and complex visual field of veridical perception is constructed from simpler elements. They are not facts about the physical world, although the neurologist can correlate them with facts known about the physical world—for instance, with the fact that there is a tumour in such and such a part of the brain. Besides, the neurologist can experience enough of these changes for himself by the use of such an agent as mescaline so as to make all this evidence relevant to our present enquiry.

10.1. The visual field presents itself to awareness, during any one specious present, as a single *spatial* and *organised* whole, in which there may be distinguished parts, visual sense-data, which are *coloured expanses*.[1] In Broad's words,[2] 'So long as it is light and one's eyes are open, one really is directly apprehending *something*, though it is not what one uncritically takes it to be. This something is an extended, spatially continuous, variously coloured and shaded field, which is presented as a finite but un-bounded whole.' The organisation and elaboration of sense-data and the actual construction of the visual field as a spatio-temporal coloured whole structure may be shown to be cor-related with the activity of a number of different mechanisms in the brain. Each of these mechanisms is correlated with a differ-ent and specific element in this process. For instance, the organ-isation of *colour* and *movement* in the field are both processes separable from the organisation of *shape*.

'The researches of the last fifty years however have shown that "seeing" in the sense of an awareness of visual sense-data is not an all-or-none process but a progressive integration and discrimination. Poppelreuter's stages have been described above. Whether or not this particular series is accepted there is ample evidence in favour of the principle.'[3]

[1] This does not *define* sense-data but only *describes* them.
[2] C. D. Broad (*c*), *Religion, Philosophy and Psychical Research*, London, 1953, p. 37.
[3] Sir Russell Brain (*b*), 'Visual object agnosia with special reference to the Gestalt theory', *Brain*, 1941, **64**, 43–62.

It is not so much the awareness that is altered in these people whose brains are in an abnormal state, but the change occurs in the actual nature of the sense-data themselves. In other words we are not dealing so much with alterations in the *sensing* of normal sense data, but with interference with the construction of the visual field.

The following account is not meant to present the whole evidence but merely those parts of it relevant to the present discussion.

10.11. *Form*. Poppelreuter's stages describe the order in which vision is regained after cerebral injuries:

'(1) The primitive Gestalt is the visual field, pure and simple, i.e. visual extension without form.

(2) In stage 2, the field becomes differentiated so that qualitatively different stimuli are experienced to left or right without form and without boundary between light and dark.

(3) Next, a surface area is differentiated but without distinct dimensions. It appears neither horizontal nor vertical, but the same dimension on all sides.

(4) In the fourth stage the mass possess a direction within the visual field.

(5) The fifth is the stage of indeterminate forms. There is a definite form differentiation, extension or dimension of the mass which is perceived as somewhat long, small, horizontal, etc.

(6) Next comes the distinction of several separate masses within the visual fields.

(7) Finally, form is perceived in the strict sense, and there is distinction of straight lines, curves, geometrical figures, etc.'[1]

An eighth stage may be described in which three-dimensional depth is added to an entirely flat picture. Gordon Holmes[2] describes a case in which this last stage is lost:

'Everything seen was flat, nothing had thickness or depth in it; stereoscopic vision was completely abolished. . . . A box seemed to him a piece of flat cardboard, no matter at what angle

[1] Brain, loc. cit., (*b*).
[2] Gordon Holmes, 'Disturbances of visual space perception', *Brit. Med. J.*, 1919, vol. 2, pp. 230–3.

he saw it, . . . And a glass tumbler looked like a piece of flat glass which changed in shape as it was moved about. When he was placed in front of a line of steps he saw only a number of straight lines on the floor.'

This change is obviously of a very different order from the relative loss of stereoscopic vision we get by closing one eye. Poppelreuter's account is possibly to some extent ideal, as no one patient shows all the stages given, but it does at least describe what may be expected if a number of such patients are studied. It illustrates the process whereby *form* is created in the visual field, the *shape* of sense-data delineated and the sense-data themselves *placed* in their sensed mutual spatial relations. Colour has its own development described below.

Another such developmental series is given by the form and behaviour of sense-data sensed by the congenitally blind restored to sight by operation. The following accounts are taken from Schilder:[1]

'Franz's patient said that three days after the operation he saw an extended field of light in which everything was dark, turned over, mixed together, and in motion; the movement later appeared as flying circles. He could not distinguish objects. . . . La Prince reports that a patient merely saw a succession of dark and light instead of a movement. . . . Beer said that patients using vision alone saw only the outlines of solid geometrical figures; for example, a sphere appeared as a circular disc, lighted more or less by single points. . . .'

Thus the visual field in these cases was at first a confused welter of light, dark, coloured, and moving sense-data which did not in the least resemble the visual field of a normal person looking at the same scene. It may be many months before a normal visual field is achieved.

10.12. *Colour and shape.* In certain lesions of the occipital lobe the phenomena of *space-colours* and *film-colours* may be encountered. Normally the colour of an object is co-extensive with its shape, but in these cases it ceases to be so. The colour

---

[1] Paul Schilder (*b*), *Mind, Perception and Thought in Their Constructive Aspects*, New York, 1942, p. 53.

may appear as a film around the shape or as a cloud in space around it. The patient will have to push his finger through this cloud to reach the object, and may exclaim in surprise at the novel experience. 'The transformation of space colour to surface colour is a part of the process of the creation of definite objects.'[1] ⟨Object⟩ here is used in the sense of Broad's 'complete optical object'.

10.13. *Movement.* The movement of sense-data or groups of sense-data making up complete optical objects may likewise be affected independently of the processes described above. Sense-data in cases of 'primitive' perception (i.e. in people with brain injuries, etc.) are often in internal movement, which movement is not exhibited by the physical object to which they belong.

'We have emphasized sufficiently that primitive perception shows motion in the majority of the sense-modalities and this inner motion is another spatial quality.'[2]

The action of mescaline may cause the sense-data belonging to physical objects to move in a rhythmical manner while the objects are stationary, and stimulation of the vestibular apparatus may also cause such movements as well as the most complex changes in the spatial interrelations of sense-data. Mescaline may also cause a moving physical object to be represented by a series of stationary sense-data strung out contemporaneously along the path which the moving sense-datum would have followed had it behaved normally.

10.14. *Spatial relations.* A fourth fundamental function which may be affected independently of the processes described above is that which determines that the spatial relations between sense-data in the visual field should be the same as those existing between the physical objects they belong to as 'viewed' or obtained, for example, by a camera at that place.[3] This function

---

[1] Paul Schilder, loc. cit. (*b*), p. 136.   [2] *Ibid.*, p. 182.

[3] Normally even this is not accurate. For psychology has shown that the complete optical object belonging to a distant material thing is *larger* than it should be according to the laws of optics. The perceptual mechanisms literally magnify distant material things suitably placed in perspective (the 'constant size' effect).

may be disturbed in a great number of ways. For instance, the visual field may be entirely inverted, or the patient may be unable to see more than two or three at any one time out of a larger number of material things presented to him. Likewise the sense-data belonging to material things may be too small (micropsia), or too big (macropsia); or seem to be 'too far away' (teleopsia), or 'too near' or only parts of them may be presented or the optical object may be fragmented and parts which are contiguous in the physical object may become widely separated and other sense-data intrude between them. The collections of sense-data making up complete optical objects may take on all manner of shapes not possessed by the physical object. Many of these changes may occur in only one half of the visual field or even only in one quarter or segment of it.

10.15. *Time.* In the phenomenon known as visual perseveration the sense-data belonging to a material thing may continue to fill their sensible positions in the visual field for quite a long time after the gaze is directed elsewhere. For instance, the patient may look at a vase on the table and then look at the mantelpiece, when the vase will be seen quite plainly to be there.

10.16. We have examples also from experimental psychology which seem to support the contention that the visual field in direct experience is built up by a representative mechanism. These are the well-known 'constant-size' effect, which shows that distant vision does not obey the physical laws of perspective and the phenomenon known as Fuchsian completions. In this, if an incomplete, though nearly complete, circle or other regular figure is presented to a subject under certain conditions, the complete figure will be sensed. If a semi-circle is presented to a subject with hemianopia so that its two horns fall just on the edge of the hemianopic field, again the complete figure will be sensed, presumably by reconstruction by the sensory mechanisms.[k]

10.17. What conclusions can we draw from all this evidence? Schilder[1] draws this one:

'We come therefore again to the general conclusion that the brain helps us to develop our undeveloped psychic material,' ...

---

[1] Paul Schilder (c), *Brain and Personality*, New York, 1951, p. 43.

Poppelreuter says that we have to deal with a number of part-systems:

'(1) the brightness system; (2) the colour system; (3) the form system; (4) movement; and (5) direction. These different part-systems may be more or less independently disturbed.'[1]

It seems reasonable to suggest that the visual field must be constructed by the representative mechanisms of our own organism. The relation R in Broad's formula o − R − s and Price's relation of *belonging to* connecting a sense-datum and the physical object it represents may be that of connection by non-symbolical representative mechanism. This hypothesis serves to link the philosophical problems of the genesis of the visual field of contiguous sense-data with the present position in neurophysiology, where the nervous system is regarded as functioning along lines similar to machines studied by communication engineers. However, in Cybernetics, the nervous system is regarded solely as a device linking the afferent sensory system to the efferent motor system. The relation of cerebral events to experiential events has not been taken into account.

Thus the visual field is not what it is because it could not possibly be anything else, or because it is literally made up by the surfaces of external physical objects. It seems to be the construction of a very complicated and most efficient mechanism.

10.2.   THE STROBOSCOPIC PATTERNS

10.21. *The facts.* The electronic stroboscope is a device in which the discharge from a condenser is passed at regular intervals through a gas-filled tube. This provides a flash of light of extremely short duration (some 10^{-5} seconds). The frequency of the flash can be varied from 1 to 40 per second. This device has been used for the last decade in electroencephalography as it was found that the electrical rhythms of the brain can be driven by the flash frequency. During this work it was noticed that when a subject looks at the flashing light certain complicated phenomena develop in his visual field. Grey Walter[1] has dis-

---

[1] Quoted by H. Klüver, *Psychol. Bull.*, 1927, **24**, 316–58.

cussed certain theoretical aspects of the phenomenon. When the light is flashed at between about 6–30 flashes per second, he will notice that his whole visual field becomes filled with complex patterns. These are usually composed of a large number of zig-zag dark or coloured lines vibrating with incessant movement upon a light ground. These lines may form a design like the spokes of a wheel or whirlpool, or catherine wheel effects may be observed. The zig-zag lines may sweep from one side of the visual field to the other. Another dominant form of the patterns is a complex mosaic of most intricate structure. Interspersed amongst these line patterns arrangements of coloured dots may be observed. At some frequencies great sheets of brilliant colours may appear and spread over the field. The actual form of the patterns observed will vary very much with the frequency of the flash and with the colour of the screen held before the eyes. A most striking feature of the phenomenon is the great complexity of the patterns.

10.22. *The interpretation of the facts.* The questions arise 'How are we to explain this phenomenon and what conclusions of philosophical interest can we draw from it?' Grey Walter[1] has suggested that the observations give us evidence that the physiological mechanisms mediating visual perception of the external world function according to the same mechanical principles as are used in television.[2] The television mechanism has three essential parts—a receptor, a conductor and a presentor. The spatio-temporal pattern of light and dark shapes (the scene televised) is transformed by the receptor into an electrical pattern of excitation conducted by wires or electromagnetic radiation. The pattern is thus transmitted to the 'set'—the presentor part of the mechanism. Here the electrical pattern is transformed by a scanning device back into a pattern similar to the original pattern televised, and thus a *copy* of the original scene is *reconstructed* by the mechanism. If the studio is illuminated by a flashing light instead of a steady light, phenomena similar to these described above—complex patterns of dots and streaks

---

[1] Grey Walter, loc. cit.

[2] It would be more correct to say that television uses the same mechanical principles as are used in the physiological mechanisms mediating visual perception.

and lines—will dart and zig-zag across the screen, because, at each flash, only that part of the screen over which the electron beam is travelling for the duration of the flash will be illuminated. The actual form of the patterns will depend on the particular nature of the scanning mechanism employed: and, therefore, if constant details of the patterns observed in the case of human vision can be recorded, we will be able to make inferences about the particular construction of the scanning mechanism responsible for them.

If a cinema studio is illuminated with a flashing light during the taking of the film, the results obtained will depend on the frequency of the flash in relation to the frame frequency of the camera. If the light flashes every time the shutter is opened, a normal film will result. If it flashes only when it is closed, the film will remain unexposed. If it flashes at a different frequency to the frame frequency of the camera, the exposures obtained will beat giving a fluctuating series of underexposed and overexposed pictures. Grey Walter[1] then describes the television process as follows:

'But in the case of the television picture the conditions are quite different [to what they are in the case of the cinema], for here each frame is scanned in the camera and the scanning is reproduced in the receiver. If the light flashes occur when the scanning beam is, say, at the top right-hand corner of the frame, then only that region will appear illuminated; if the frequencies of frame and flicker differ slightly, the bright spot of illumination will appear to drift or dart over the screen—that is, an illusion of movement can be generated by the combination of a flickering light and a scanning generator. . . . In other words, the televisual system behaves very much like the neuro-visual one.'

'Perhaps the most interesting of these observations is the chequered appearance of the visual field and the violent movement of its separate elements, since this is precisely what one would expect to see if a scanning rhythm were attempting to transform an excitation field uniformly stimulated at a frequency similar to that of the scanning rhythm itself.'

'. . . a large intermittent signal of this sort is precisely what one would use to jam an artificial device which included a scanning

---

[1] Grey Walter, loc. cit., pp. 77, 74 and 76.

system, because not only would any other signal be masked; an entirely spurious set of messages would appear *on the far side of the scanner.*' (My italics.)

Now the following points may be noted:

10.221. The sensed visual patterns comprising the stroboscopic phenomena are quite flat and two-dimensional. They have no visual depth. They are *spatial* patterns and fill the entire visual field—as far to the right and left, above and below as one can direct one's attention. The patterns are spatially located, it would seem, about two feet in front of the (sensed) nose. That is to say they are located where after-images are located.

10.222. Secondly, from the (direct) observation of these patterns it is possible to make certain suggestions about the nature of the physiological processes mediating everyday visual perception. The stroboscopic phenomena which may be observed on the screen of the ordinary television set when we interfere in a specific way with the workings of the mechanism, do not arise *de novo* but owe their origin to the fact that the mechanism which presents the 'normal' pictures on the television screen is constructed in a particular way. The images we ordinarily see on the screen of the set are themselves constructed by the same scanning mechanism when it is functioning without such interference. Similarly the complex patterns we observe when our own physiological mechanisms of perception are subjected to intermittent stimulation do not arise *de novo,* but they suggest that the expanded and coloured visual field as this presents itself to direct observation is itself *constructed* by the physiological mechanisms mediating visual perception, and thus the visual field cannot be a structural part of the 'external world'. For as we sit in front of the stroboscope with our eyes shut[1] watching the intricate play of the stroboscopic patterns we can argue as follows:

'When my eyes are directed at this flashing light the patterns that I see suggest that what I directly observe is a (spatial) field in which the events are being immediately determined by a most complex and intricate scanning device. Now, when I look away from the lamp at the scene around illuminated by a steady light,

---

[1] The lids function as a red semi-opaque filter.

I can no longer detect these patterns. My field of direct observation is now filled with (relatively) stable and contiguous patches of colour (sense-data). Nevertheless it is evident that this complex pattern of shaped colours must, if this hypothesis is true, be built up by the individual elements demonstrated by the stroboscopic process. For the stroboscopic stimulation can only reveal the details of the mode of construction of the visual field. The representative mechanism is designed not to produce curious patterns when the receptor part of the mechanism is illuminated by a flashing light, but to construct a *copy* of the scene at which the receptor part of the mechanism is directed under normal conditions of illumination. That is to say that, when I look at a scene illuminated with a steady light, the position and form and colour of each and every minute element in the whole visual field[1] is determined by the physiological mechanisms of perception functioning as representative mechanisms constructing a *copy* of the scene at which my receptor sensory organs (eyes) are directed. I cannot suppose that I have one entire physiological mechanism mediating my visual perception of scenes illuminated by a flashing light and another to mediate my perception of scenes illuminated by a steady light, which second mechanism might be supposed to use different physiological principles which might be said to give me a *direct* view of the external physical world—of the scene before my receptor sensory organs—without the mediation of any such *copy* or *representation* of the scene. For it is mechanically impossible for the televisual mechanism (or any other mechanism) to give us a direct view of the events televised or represented. The stroboscopic phenomena suggest that my perception of scenes illuminated by the stroboscopic lamp, and so of all scenes illuminated by an ordinary light, is mediated by a televisual mechanism. As Grey Walter[2] says, "The televisual mechanism behaves very much like the neuro-visual one." '

It is however possible that the stroboscopic patterns originate in the complex mechanism of the retina. In which case we

[1] A *visual field* contains only sense-data: the term ⟨field of vision⟩ is used to denote those physical objects materially and functionally present to the external sense organs.

[2] Grey Walter, loc. cit., p. 76.

can postulate a static *point-to-point* projection (and not a scanning projection) from the visual cortex to the visual field to complete the causal chain of perception on its afferent side. This point-to-point connection may be thought of as similar in principle to the point-to-point projection linking the retina to the cortex. The patterns may also derive partly from the retinal mechanism and partly from scanning mechanisms farther along the causal chain mediating perception, i.e. in the cerebral cortex or in the processes connecting the cortex to the visual field. Experimental work is at present in progress to determine which of these alternatives is correct. It should be noted that one of the basic postulates of this theory is that the physiological mechanisms of perception are representative mechanisms which actually construct the visual field of contiguous sense-data. It is of secondary importance whether this construction is affected by a scanning mechanism or by a point-to-point causal relation. In either case we should be able to determine something of interest about the mechanisms of perception from a detailed study of the stroboscopic patterns.[m]

10.223. Could we perhaps say that the stroboscopic phenomena indicate only that there are scanning mechanisms in the sensory parts of the cortex? However, stroboscopic patterns related to, or produced by, a scanning mechanism must always be an integral *part*[1] of the mechanism. The sensed stroboscopic patterns in human vision are sensibly located *outside* the sensed skull (in which phenomenalist and naïve realist theories *locate* the physical brain) and therefore cannot be *in* the brain (under these theories). Even if there are scanning mechanisms in the brain, the stroboscopic patterns witnessed on looking at a flashing light cannot literally be parts of, nor can they be constructed by, these mechanisms, for not only are they spatially external to the somatic sensory field (which is identified in phenomenalist and naïve realist theories with the physical organism), but they are non-congruent with, and thus cannot be identical with, any schema (pattern of neuronal activity) in the brain. And if it is

---

[1] In the sense that the images on a television screen are a part of the television mechanism, although, of course, not in the sense that one of the valves is a part of this mechanism.

said that the sensed patterns are 'really' in the occipital cortex and only 'seem' to be outside, we can ask what are the neurophysiological processes underlying this process whereby patterns of neuronal activity 'seem' to be spatially located outside the organism and, moreover, appear as totally different patterns to any found in the brain. The phenomenalist and naïve realist, it appears, might have to say that there are processes concerned in perception which have no neurophysiological basis, for I do not know what neurophysiological process there could be whereby neurophysiological processes themselves would seem to themselves—or to other neurophysiological processes —to be located outside the organism altogether.

Chapter Three

THE STATUS OF SOMATIC
SENSE-DATA

---

11. THERE is always present in a man's direct experience an entity which he naïvely, unreflectingly, unquestioningly thinks of as *my body*, or, if he is more sophisticated, as *my physical body*, or even *my organism*. This entity is composed of the totality of all somatic sense-data available to inspection (in Broad's sense) in any specious present. In neurology this entity is usually mis-called the *body-image* or sometimes the *body-schema*, and in common sense it is regarded quite simply as being the physical body. This is however a mistake. As Hutton[1] says:

'The difficulty of both realists and idealists seems to arise from a confusion of the perceived body [somatic sense-data] with the percipient's actual body. Because of the experienced dependency of all perceived objects upon the perceived state of the percipient's body the ability to perceive them is located within this perceived body, and the mind is thought of as being located within this perceived skull; but what is often forgotten is that this body and this skull are themselves objects of perception.'

[1] Hutton, in Richter (ed.) loc. cit., p. 156: ⟨sense⟩ is better here than ⟨perceive⟩.

And Schilder:[1]

'But the empirical method leads immediately to a deep insight that even our own body is beyond our immediate reach, that even our own body justifies Prospero's words: "We are such stuff as dreams are made on; and our little life is rounded with a sleep." '

And Köhler:[2]

'I learned that physical objects influence a particularly interesting physical system, my organism [physical body], and that my objective experience results when, as a consequence, certain complicated processes have happened in this system. Obviously, I realised, I cannot identify the final products, the things and events of my experience [sense-data], with the physical objects from which the influences come. If a wound is not the gun which emitted the projectile, then the things which I have before me, which I see and feel [visual and tactile sense-data] cannot be identical with the corresponding physical objects. These objects merely establish certain alterations within my physical organism [physical body], and the final products of these alterations are the things which I behold in my visual field [visual sense-data], or which I feel with my fingers [tactual sense-data]. We have seen that the same warning applies to the relation between my organism as a physical system and my body as a perceptual fact [sensed body or somatic sensory field]. My body [sensed body] is the outcome of certain processes in my physical organism, processes which start in the eyes, muscles, skin and so forth, exactly as the chair before me [visual sense-data belonging to the chair] is the final product of other processes in the same physical organism. If the chair is seen "before me", the "me" of this phrase means my body as an experience [sensed body], of course, not my organism as an object of the physical world. Even psychologists do not always seem to be entirely clear about this point.'

In the theory of naïve realism no distinction would be drawn between the sensed body and the physical body. There is just *the body, my body*—my alleged direct experience of my own physi-

[1] Paul Schilder (*d*), *The Image and Appearance of the Human Body*, London, 1935, p. 304.
[2] Wolfgang Köhler, *Gestalt Psychology*, New York, 1947, p. 22.

76

cal organism. The phenomenon rather misleadingly named the *phantom limb* is enough to invalidate this view. If the physical limb is amputated, or if there is any sufficiently drastic interference with the sensory pathway from the limb as in the case of a cord tumour, the somatic sense-data very often continue to be sensed and these are qualitatively indistinguishable from those sensed before the operation or development of the tumour. The 'phantom limb' is nothing *new* but is composed of familiar somatic sense-data. It does not behave as it did before of course, but it can nevertheless often be *moved* voluntarily and shows the phenomenon of associated movements, and may be felt to itch, sweat, flush or tingle, often in appropriate situations. In some cases of spinal cord lesions the whole lower half of the somatic sensory field will continue to be sensed, often in a position different to that taken up by the physical body at the time, in spite of the interruption of the sensory pathway. Thus it is clear that somatic sense-data cannot literally be parts of the physical body, since the physical limb in these amputation cases has long since been incinerated or lies pickled in a specimen jar. Thus the theory of naïve realism will not hold even when applied to that most intimate of physical objects—my physical body.

This conclusion has been obscured in neurology by the current confusion over the use of the term ⟨body-image⟩. This has been used to describe a number of quite different entities, i.e. (11.1) the *sensed body*, (11.2) the *body concept*, and (11.3) the *body schema*.

11.1. We have described the *sensed body* above. It corresponds to Wisdom's *phantom body*. A clear case in neurology of the use of the term ⟨body-image⟩ to denote it may be found in Macdonald Critchley:[1]

'In such conditions [in cases where there was an imperception for one half of the body], the most plausible explanation of these cases of tactile allochiria is to imagine a unilateral defect of the body-image, without, however, absolute sensory loss. A pinprick applied to the affected side is felt, but it is not accurately projected, that particular half of the body-image being in

[1] Macdonald Critchley (*a*), *The Parietal Lobes*, London, 1953, pp. 138 and 240.

abeyance.   It is therefore naturally transferred to a corresponding point on the intact half of the body-image.'

And again:

'With the onset of this vision, the feeling of strangeness of the left half of his body-image disappeared.'

Critchley had previously defined the body-image as:[1] 'the mental idea which an individual possesses as to his body and its physical and aesthetic attributes'; i.e. the body concept. But a mental idea does not have spatial halves, nor is it concerned with sensory localisation, nor can an idea *feel* strange. ⟨Body-image⟩ here clearly denotes the somatic sensory field.

I will give one more example out of the many to be found in the literature:[2]

'Federn has made some excellent observations and analyses of the changes that take place in the body-image during the stage of falling asleep. . . . Two phenomena belong especially to this group; the first are the changes in the sensory evaluation of the magnitude of particular parts of the body; for example, the extremities, the head, parts of the face become disproportionately large or small; . . .'

These changes take place in the sensed body and no changes in the body concept are involved.

11.2. Secondly we all possess a system of concepts, of knowledge, beliefs, wishes, attitudes, etc., about our own physical bodies and those of other people. We know, for example, that we have two legs and two arms, a tubular shape, the colour of our hair, eyes, etc. We can call this conceptual constellation—the *body-concept*. People with phantom limbs experience the puzzling phantom limb but they are not persuaded by it that they 'really' do have the physical limb which they feel but which they know has gone. Thus they have no disorder of their body-concepts. Yet some hemiplegics deny the possession of their hemiplegic limb and others believe that they have a number of

---

[1] Macdonald Critchley (*b*), *Lancet*, 1950, **258**, 335–40.
[2] G. Bychowski, 'Disorders in the body-image in the clinical picture of psychoses', *J. Nerv. Ment. Dis.*, 1943, **97**, 310–35.

supernumerary limbs—Weinstein[1] has recently reported a number of such cases. These people do have disorders of their body-concepts—well-marked delusions in fact—as well as their disorders of sensation. Beliefs and knowledge are different from sensations yet the current use of the term ⟨body-image⟩ confuses them beyond repair.

11.3. Thirdly there is the *body-schema*. The term ⟨body-schema⟩ is often wrongly used where (1) or (2) should be used. This was introduced by Head and Holmes and should be used in their original sense to describe a purely physiological mechanism:[2]

'But, in addition to its function as an organ for local attention, the sensory cortex is also the storehouse of past impressions. These may rise into consciousness as images, but more often, as in the case of spacial impressions, remain outside central consciousness. Here they form organised models of ourselves which may be termed "schemata". Such schemata modify the impressions produced by incoming sensory impulses in such a way that the final sensations of position, or of locality, rise into consciousness charged with a relation to something that has happened before.'

It may be noticed that, taking the Self as central, the physical body is on the distal side of this charging process; that the body-schema is at the site of the charging process and that the sensed body is on its proximal side. The experiments of Stratton *et al.* (quoted by Schilder[3]) give a good example of how an almost pure disorder of the body-schemata may be built up by feeding them with contradictory sensory information.

11.4. Lastly there are true *body-images*. These are merely ordinary mental images representing a human body.

11.5. Now unless we differentiate between all these clearly it becomes difficult to distinguish between (1) and the physical body. For if we confuse (1) and (2), the question 'what is the relation between the body-image and the physical organism?'

---

[1] E. A. Weinstein *et al.*, 'Delusional reduplication of parts of the body', *Brain*, 1954, **77**, 45–60.

[2] H. Head and G. Holmes, 'Sensory disturbances from cerebral lesions', *Brain*, 1911, **34**, 102–254.

[3] Schilder, loc. cit. (*d*), pp. 108–12.

becomes the question of the relation of a concept or conceptual constellation to the physical organism. But if we distinguish clearly between (1) and (2), we can ask 'what is the relation between the somatic sensory field and the physical organism?' and use evidence from neurology couched in body-image terminology as relevant. Wisdom went right to the root of the problem in the concluding passage in his address to the 11th International Philosophical Congress:[1]

'Nonetheless there are merits about such an identification [to call the phantom-body a mind]. It would suggest that the problem of mind-body dualism centres around the relation between the phantom-body and the physiological body, and that the relations between the phantom-body, attitude system, and perceptual and reflective consciousness constitute a problem in the domain of psychology.'

But he does not make it quite clear in this paper that a 'phantom body' is, for you and me, the oh-so-familiar collection of somatic sense-data that form the ever-present background to (waking) experience. We do not experience the physiological body normally and have latent a phantom body ready to manifest parts of itself only when there is an amputation or a suitable neurological lesion in the physical body. We never experience directly the physiological body at all: we merely (mistakenly) identify the somatic sensory field with it (in 'commonsense') and then are surprised when we do not lose parts of the somatic sensory field when we lose (or lose touch with) corresponding parts of the physical body. We have mistaken a causal relation (e.g. of mechanical coupling) for an ontological identity.

[1] J. O. Wisdom, 'The concept of "phantom-body" ', *Proc. XIth Int. Cong. Phil.*, 1953, **7**, 175–9.

Chapter Four

VERIDICAL
AND HALLUCINATORY
SENSE-EXPERIENCE

12. HALLUCINATORY sense-perception has been a perennial puzzle to philosophers of perception. For, if we think that, in ordinary sense-experience, we experience physical objects directly and that there are no other entities in the universe besides physical objects, we must hold that hallucinations are 'unreal'. But hallucinatory experience is qualitatively indistinguishable, in many cases, from veridical sense-experience. Hallucinations are spatial and coloured entities and may possess not only a high degree of internal organisation, but may also be closely integrated into the 'veridical' remainder of the visual field in which they occur. Furthermore people who are actually having hallucinatory experiences under optimal conditions (i.e. when they are not also confused, insane or ill) frequently cannot be persuaded that their experiences are in any sense unreal. At least that is our experience in the large number of experiments that we have conducted giving hallucinogenic agents to ordinary and (philosophically) sophisticated people. The experiences are regarded as not 'unreal' but different. In some cases, on the other hand, a state of derealisation may be produced by these

agents. This may also occur in the course of a psychiatric illness. In such a case the person will complain that the ordinary world 'looks unreal'. Derealisation is a specific disorder of perception in which the visual field loses its normal 'concrete reality' and everything appears vague, shadowy, distant, indifferent, unreal. In contrast some of the mescaline phenomena have a very lively reality, using reality in the same sense that the visual field of the person who is derealised may be said to have lost its reality. Thus the factors which determine whether ordinary people call their experiences real or unreal do not necessarily depend on whether the experiences are veridical or hallucinatory. It depends more upon the particular quality of the experience. Both veridical and hallucinatory experiences may be regarded as being real or unreal. In any case the puzzle remains—how can any spatial and highly organised entity be unreal?

Ayer says that the reason why we pronounce our dream experiences and other hallucinatory experiences to be delusive is because[1] 'they do not fit into the general order of our experience', and again[2] 'For the only way in which one can test whether a series of perceptions is veridical, in this sense, is to see whether it is substantiated by further sense experiences'; 'so that once again the ascription of "reality" depends on the predictive value of the sense-data on which the perceptions are based'. But this assumes that there is only one 'general order' to our experiences whereas in fact there are two such orders. Ayer, in these passages, is laying down criteria for the use of the word ⟨real⟩. These criteria function very well for the ordinary biological processes of living. They may prevent us from setting off into the waterless desert in pursuit of a miraged oasis or from throwing our shoes at an hallucinatory cat. But they do not fit the sensible facts properly. For the same criteria that Ayer uses to distinguish between hallucinatory and veridical sense-experience may be used to classify hallucinatory sense-experience itself. Ayer's criteria for determining the 'reality' of a sense-experience are (i) that it must fit into the general order of our experience, and (ii) that it must be substantiated by further sense-experiences. It must be noted that ⟨it⟩ in the first

[1] Ayer, loc. cit., p. 42. [2] *Ibid.*, p. 274.

criterion denotes the *order* of the experiences to be substantiated and not any particular sense-experience itself. That is to say 'to substantiate a series of perceptions' means 'to sense a further series of sense-data which must come within the general order, in certain specified ways, of the previous set of sense-experiences to be substantiated'.

12.1. But before this argument can be further developed I will give a brief account of hallucinations as they occur in nature. A preliminary classification (which will be replaced later when it has served its introductory purpose) may be made as follows:

(i) Hallucinations of a trivial nature which occur in normal people.

(ii) Hallucinations of a more complex nature which occur in normal people.

(iii) Hallucinations which occur in cases of abnormality of the nervous system.

(iv) The mescaline phenomena to which the hypnagogic phenomena are closely allied.

To consider these in more detail:

(i) Into this class fall such trivial events as the example given by Price of seeing a 9 instead of a 6 on a number 6 bus when we are hopefully awaiting the arrival of a number 9 bus. Another example is the case recorded by Miss Jephson[1] of the occasion when she saw a cheque in her purse when there was really not one there at all. Such trivial hallucinations are easily induced in susceptible subjects by hypnosis.

(ii) More complex hallucinatory experiences can also occur in quite normal people as the *Census of Hallucinations*[2] clearly showed. Examples include the so-called 'apparitions' of living and dead people, the Moberly case,[3] the Dieppe raid case[4] and the more complex hallucinations induced by hypnosis.[5] It is

[1] Ina Jephson, 'An interesting hallucination', *J. Soc. Psychical Research*, 1932, **27**, 184.

[2] Sidgwick *et al.*, 'The census of hallucinations', *Proc. Soc. Psychical Research*, 1894, **10**, 25–422.

[3] C. A. E. Moberly and E. F. Jourdain, *An Adventure*, London, 1911.

[4] G. W. Lambert and Kathleen Gay, 'The Dieppe raid case', *J. Soc. Psychical Research*, 1952, **36**, 607–18.

[5] Ian Fletcher, 'Recent experiments in hypnotism', *J. Soc. Psychical Research*, 1949, **35**, 101–8.

characteristic of such hallucinations that the hallucinatory sense-data are well integrated into the veridical remainder of the visual field in which they occur. In most of the descriptions recorded the hallucinated person appears perfectly solid, throws a shadow, gets smaller as he moves away from the observer, moves around the room with respect for the furniture, etc. (Tyrrell's account should be consulted for further details.)[1] Thus it is an empirical fact that hallucinations experienced by normal people show various degrees of organisation and complexity. They may be quite fleeting and trivial, or the hallucinated figure may fit so well into the veridical remainder of the visual field that some time may elapse before the observer realises that he is confronted with an hallucination and not a living person. In the case of apparitions the true nature of the experience is usually revealed when the apparition, after behaving in a 'normal' fashion for a time, suddenly drifts through a wall or disappears while in full view. Yet the organisation possessed by this class of experience is in general the same as that possessed by veridical sense-experience. In fact it is because apparitions frequently look so like and behave so like living people that they are so frequently confused with them. Thus such a series of hallucinatory experiences as those reported by Tyrrell only just fail to belong to the general order of our experience. That is to say that some members of the total series do, for a while, belong to the order of veridical sense-experience, but this membership is cancelled by a subsequent experience. Whereas hallucinations of class (iv) never belong to this order at all.

(iii) A great variety of hallucinations may be found in various medical conditions and these vary in their degree and type of organisation and to the degree to which they are or are not integrated with the veridical remainder of the visual field. But they form only an intermediate stage between the hallucinations of normal people which, as they become more complex, tend to become increasingly well integrated into the veridical remainder of the field in which they occur, and the hallucinations of type (iv), which, as they become more complex, tend to attain quite a different organisation to that of the ordinary visual field. We can therefore pass directly to the fourth class of hallucination.

[1] G. N. M. Tyrrell, *Apparitions*, London, 1953.

(iv) Mescaline,[1] a vegetable alkaloid, is found in nature in the juices of a small Mexican desert cactus, *Anhalonium Lewinii*. The Mexican desert Indians prepare a brew, *peyotl*, from the plant and use this for their religious ceremonies. Scattered references to this practice may be found in the writings of the Spanish Jesuit priests of the seventeenth century. It was only discovered for Western science in 1886 by the great pharmacologist, Lewin, after whom the cactus is named. His reports aroused a certain amount of interest at the time, and a number of investigators carried out research into its action. Weir Mitchell and Havelock Ellis were among the most notable of these.[2] A second wave of interest in the drug was aroused by the publication in 1927 of Beringer's and Rouhier's monographs.[3] Since then mescaline has been used chiefly by psychiatrists who have taken it to undergo themselves something of the experiences of their schizophrenic patients.[4] Rouhier, indeed, hoped that the drug would be of use in psychoanalysis, and Havelock Ellis expressed the opinion that a drug with such marvellous effects would soon become popular. But neither of these hopes have been realised, and this extraordinary substance remains in almost complete obscurity.

Mescaline has quite a simple chemical formula and it is thought to work by interfering with the action of an enzyme in the brain which consequently becomes unable to use glucose properly. When taken by a normal subject it produces marked changes in perception, sensation, feeling, in some cases thinking, and in the relation between the ego and its environment, some of which changes are so remarkable as to defy description. It produces varied effects in different subjects, and the following account represents what may be expected to happen if a number of subjects are chosen. Each will experience in varying degree

[1] This section is reprinted from the *British Journal for the Philosophy of Science*, 1953, **3**, 339–47, with a few changes.

[2] S. Weir Mitchell, 'Remarks on the effects of Anhalonium Lewinii', *Brit. Med. J.*, 1896, **2**, 1625–9, and Havelock Ellis, 'Mescal. A new artificial paradise', *Ann. Rep. Smithsonian Institute*, 1897, I, 537–48.

[3] A. Rouhier, *Le Peyotl*, Paris, 1927, and K. Beringer, *Mescalinrausch*, Berlin, 1927.

[4] H. Osmond and J. Smythies, 'Schizophrenia. A new approach', *J. Ment. Sci.*, 1952, **98**, 309–15.

some different combination of the totality of possible effects. None will experience them all. A few will experience only a minimal reaction. There appears to be a correlation between the quality of the experiences and the personality of the subject. The unexpected features of the mescaline phenomena are, to make my point briefly, that the hallucinations or visions it produces are often of surpassing beauty and possess the utmost poetical integrity.

Some two hours after taking mescaline the subject will begin to see, if he keeps his eyes closed, vague patches of colour floating about in his visual field. These soon develop into more complex sensa: mosaics, networks, flowing arabesques, interlaced spirals, wonderful tapestries, and patterns and designs of all sorts, all swiftly coming and going and all in the most beautiful colours and exquisite design. Then formed objects appear, great butterflies gently moving their wings, fields of glittering jewels, silver birds flying through silver forests, golden fountains and golden rain, masks, statues, fabulous animals, soaring architecture, gardens, cities, and finally human figures and fully formed scenes where coherent histories are enacted. If the subject opens his eyes the colours of objects become much more intense, deep, rich, and glowing, and they change their shape in curious and pleasing ways. One of my subjects, a highly intelligent and level-headed doctor, spent a quarter of an hour gazing at a plain glass full of water and trying to describe to me the perfection of its diamond brilliance. I myself was astounded by the heightened sparkle and glow of a wonderful mellow inner light that some wine-glasses in a cabinet developed. One curious feature of this change is that it appears to be somewhat selective. Some objects become more beautiful than others. These are most likely to be the sort of simple object that a painter would choose to paint as a still life. An artistically worthless picture in a cheap magazine remains as ugly as ever, even though its colours may become richer.

These effects may not be explained by supposing that the subject is mentally deranged or 'drunk', as in most cases it is clear that he is perfectly normal in these respects. There is commonly no interference with the powers of careful observation and objective reporting. These inspected events are quite simply extremely beautiful. Everyone who has taken mescaline will make it plain that it is necessary to experience these phenomena one-self in order fully to understand them, and to realise that all the superlatives that may be used in an attempt to describe them are miserably inadequate. Having given that warning, let me present the following extracts from the accounts of the various investigators.

From Prentiss and Morgan:[1]

'Then followed a train of delightful visions such as no human being ever enjoyed under normal conditions. My mind was perfectly clear and active; the power to concentrate my thoughts upon any desired subject was only slightly lessened; seated at my desk, I could write of my sensations and experiences; stretched out upon the bed, with closed eyes, an ever-changing panorama of infinite beauty and grandeur, of infinite variety of colour and form, hurried before me.'

From Weir Mitchell:[2]

'The display which, for an enchanted two hours followed, was such as I find it quite hopeless to describe in language which shall convey to others the beauty and splendour of what I saw . . .'
'A white spear of grey stone grew up to a huge height and became a tall, richly finished Gothic tower of very elaborate and definite design, with many rather worn statues standing in the doorways or on stone brackets. As I gazed every projecting angle, cornice, and even the face of the stones at their joinings were by degrees covered or hung with clusters of what seemed to be huge precious stones, but uncut, some being like masses of transparent fruit. . . . All seemed to possess an interior light, and to give the faintest idea of the perfectly satisfying intensity and purity of these gorgeous colour-fruits is quite beyond my power. All the colours I have ever beheld are dull as compared to these. As I looked, and it lasted long, the tower became a fine mouse hue, and everywhere the vast pendant masses of emerald green, ruby reds, and orange began to drip a slow rain of colours. . . . After an endless display of less beautiful marvels I saw that which deeply impressed me. An edge of a huge cliff

[1] D. W. Prentiss and F. P. Morgan, 'Anhalonium Lewinii (Mescal Buttons)', *Therap. Gazette*, 1895, **9**, 577–85.
[2] S. Weir Mitchell, loc. cit.

seemed to project over a gulf of unseen depth. My viewless enchanter set on the brink a huge bird claw of stone. Above from the stem or leg hung a fragment of some stuff. This began to unroll and float out to a distance which seemed to me to represent Time as well as immensity of Space. Here were miles of rippled purples, half transparent, and of ineffable beauty. Now and then soft golden clouds floated from these folds, or a great shimmer went over the whole of the rolling purples, and things, like green birds, fell from it, fluttering down into the gulf below. Next I saw clusters of stones hanging down in masses, from the claw toes, as it seemed to me miles of them down far below into the underworld of the black gulf.'

From Havelock Ellis:[1]

'The visions never resembled familiar objects; they were extremely definite, yet always novel; they were constantly approaching, and yet constantly eluding the semblance of known things. I would see thick, glorious fields of jewels, solitary or clustered, sometimes brilliant and sparkling, sometimes with a dull rich glow. Then they would spring up into flowerlike shapes beneath my gaze, and then seem to turn into gorgeous butterfly forms or endless folds of glistening, iridescent, fibrous wings of wonderful insects; while sometimes I seemed to be gazing into a vast hollow revolving vessel, on whose polished concave mother-of-pearl surface the hues were swiftly changing. I was surprised, not only by the enormous profusion of the imagery presented to my gaze, but still more by its variety. Perpetually some totally new kind of effect would appear in the field of vision: sometimes there was swift movement, sometimes dull, sombre richness of colour, sometimes glitter and sparkle, once a startling rain of gold, which seemed to approach me. . . . I was further impressed, not only by the brilliance, delicacy, and variety of the colours, but even more by their lovely and various textures—fibrous, woven, polished, glowing, dull, veined, semi-transparent. . . .'

From Knauer and Maloney:[2]

' . . . high above me, is a dome of the most beautiful mosaics, a vision of all that is most gorgeous and harmonious in colour.

[1] Havelock Ellis, loc. cit.
[2] A. Knauer and W. J. M. A. Maloney, 'A preliminary note on the psychic action of mescaline', *J. Nerv. Ment. Dis.*, 1913, **40**, 397–413.

The prevailing tint is blue, but the multitude of shades, each of such wonderful individuality, make me feel that hitherto I have been totally ignorant of what the word colour really means. The colour is intensely beautiful, rich, deep, deep, deep, wonderfully deep blue. It is like the blue of the mosque of Omar in Jerusalem. . . . A beautiful palace, filled with rare tapestries, pictures, and Louis Quinze furniture has been peacefully unfolding itself, room after room, each a little different from all the rest, all marvellously bright and beautiful, and all coloured in the same scheme—violet, cream, and gold.'

From Rouhier:[1]

'It is night—water—yet more water—always with the reflection of the moon. It is wonderful to see. A great expanse of water on which a long galley is gliding—a young girl is standing on its prow. An unseen light is flooding it with brilliant mauve beams following the movement of the boat. The water is spattered with mauve reflections—the violet glimmer plays on the white sails of a fleet of accompanying galleys. . . .'

'The sombre porch of a church before which is standing an old woman in white. A monk comes out of the church followed by a young girl also in white. He carries a lantern which lights up all three. Their movements are slow and majestic. They each have an amazing personality. This little picture is inexpressible in depth of meaning and expression. It is an illuminated and living sculpture.'

This subject subsequently described her experience thus: that she had received 'an experience of unimaginable art, unforgettable, and of an intensity for which there are no words and which it is necessary to experience in order to understand'.

From Klüver:[2]

'. . . it is true that the experiences in the mescal state are not easily forgotten. One looks "beyond the horizon" of the normal world, and this "beyond" is often so impressive or even shocking that its after-effects linger for years in one's memory.'

---

[1] A. Rouhier, *Le Peyotl*, Paris, 1927 (my own translation).

[2] H. Klüver, *Mescal, The Divine Plant and its Psychological Effects*, London, 1928, pp. 105–6.

Veridical and Hallucinatory Sense-Experience

From Havelock Ellis:[1]

'. . . a large part of its charm lies in the halo of beauty which it casts round the simplest and commonest things. . . . If it should ever chance that the consumption of mescal becomes a habit, the favourite poet of the mescal drinker will certainly be Words-worth. Not only the general attitude of Wordsworth, but many of his most memorable poems and phrases can not—one is almost tempted to say—be appreciated in their full significance by one who has never been under the influence of mescal.'

From Macdonald Critchley:[2]

'The usual emotional content of the hallucinosis is best described as one of amazement, awe, interest, and delight. The character of the visions is such as to impress the most prosaic and unimaginative scientific observer in a manner of which no natural beauty or grandeur is capable. Almost all writers have insisted that the most skilful pen or brush could not do justice to the marvel of the hallucinations.'

Changes may also be produced in other senses. Auditory hallucinations of wonderful music and voices speaking in strange languages have been reported but are rare. The sensed body may undergo the most extraordinary changes; parts may grow or shrivel, become stone-heavy and cold; the sensed limbs may detach themselves from the body and lie on the floor beside the observer. This latter effect may strike an onlooker as being amusing since the subject's physical limbs are clearly in their proper place. This amusement does not survive the onlooker's own experience of this phenomenon. Touch and pressure sense may also be affected and hard objects may be felt to be soft and malleable. An irresistible desire then arises to engage in the novel experience of moulding stones and kneading the walls of the room. Fragrant perfumes may be smelt and curious tastes experienced. Finally, in the realm of sensation, the in-teresting phenomenon of synaesthesia may occur. Sounds may be accompanied by 'appropriate' visual imagery, as may emo-tions, but the process sometimes goes further than this and

[1] Havelock Ellis, loc. cit.

[2] Macdonald Critchley (c), 'Some forms of drug addiction. Mescalism', *Brit. J. Inebriety*, 1931, **28**, 99–108.

forms of perception intermediate between the various senses may be experienced. The subject may, for example, be quite unable to say whether his experience is visual or auditory. Schilder[1] believes that such synaesthesiae represent very primitive forms of sense perception.

This account of the mescaline phenomena makes it clear that the order that they possess is a different order from that possessed by veridical perception and by the hallucinations of the first two classes. The hallucinations of class (iv) do not occur as 'wild' sense-data integrated into an otherwise normal visual field. They are seen mainly with the eyes shut and are not integrated with the ordinary visual field at all, but are quite apart from it. When the eyes are open they usually disappear or form a faint background to the veridical visual field. In other cases they may be noticed in the visual field, but in this case the visual field will itself be changed. Sometimes the entire visual field obtained with the eyes open will be replaced by (or filled with) hallucinatory sense-data. The order that the mescaline phenomena possess is characterised by extreme delicacy of form and colour, by the extreme beauty and poetical integrity of each hallucinated pattern, design, object, scene or panorama and by their ever-changing variety. The visual field obtained with the eyes open may, under mescal, take on these qualities of beauty and intense poetical value far in excess of any such qualities that the same scene may possess under ordinary circumstances.

12.2. Thus it is true to say that ordinary sense-experience has an order and that any sense-experience can only be judged to be veridical or hallucinatory in Ayer's sense by seeing if it belongs to *this* order. But that is not to say that hallucinatory sense-experience does not possess any order at all. Hallucinations of types (i) and (ii) and some of those of type (iii) are ordered to various degrees like (but always to a lesser degree than) veridical sense-experience whereas hallucinations of type (iv) possess an order of a different kind.

Furthermore, while we are having a series of hallucinatory experiences we can certainly make predictions from them which can be confirmed by further hallucinatory sense-experiences.

[1] P. Schilder, loc. cit. (*b*).

For instance, I may be watching the continuous kaleidoscopic display that we witness if we shut our eyes some hours after taking a dose of mescaline. If I consider any one such complex hallucination—it might be an incomparably lovely garden—I cannot make the particular predictions that I could make if I were looking at an ordinary garden in the physical world but I can certainly make others. I can say 'this scene will shortly be replaced by another one' and, as empirical observation has shown, this prediction will very probably be confirmed by my subsequent hallucinatory sense-experience. For a constant feature of the mescaline phenomena is that the patterns, scenes, designs, etc. witnessed are always changing. We have come across no case in our experiments,[1] nor in the extensive literature on this subject, where the hallucinatory experience has consisted throughout of only one scene or pattern. In certain instances it is even possible to predict what kind of scene will replace the one I am now looking at. For instance, if one flash of the stroboscopic lamp is directed at my closed eyes, I will notice that the complex hallucinated pattern will immediately change to be replaced by a more primitive pattern.[2] It is not necessary to suppose that, in order to establish the 'reality' of hallucinatory sense-experience, we have to be able to make from one set of hallucinatory sense-data predictions which would require a subsequent series of veridical sense-experiences to verify the predictions and so substantiate the phenomena, nor vice versa, although this can be done at times to a very limited extent. For instance, I can make a prediction when I see a large object approaching my head rapidly that I may shortly 'see stars'. Similarly on occasions hallucinatory sense-experiences have been alleged to be veridical as in the case of alleged veridical apparitions of the recently dead and of alleged precognitive dreams such as the series described by J. W. Dunne.[3] Such predictions are not biologically useful but their empirical and logical status is not the wit impaired by that. If we qualify

[1] Conducted in association with Dr. Humphrey Osmond and Edward Osborn, Esq.

[2] D. Peretz, J. R. Smythies and W. C. Gibson, 'A New Hallucinogen', *J. Ment. Sci.*, 1955, **101,** 317–29.

[3] J. W. Dunne, *An Experiment with Time*, London, 1927.

Ayer's criteria to admit only what is of biological survival value to the organism we have only defined what is 'biologically' real. We cannot however assume that what is real in the universe is necessarily only that which is biologically useful to man. Thus we cannot classify experience into two watertight classes real and delusive using Ayer's criteria. Such a method yields only grades of 'reality'.

The order exhibited by hallucinatory sense-data of type (iv) is inferior, in one sense, to that exhibited by veridical sense-data, in that the predictions we can make from the former are much more limited than those we can make from the latter. But, in another aspect of the concept of order, the mescaline phenomena possess a much higher degree of order than does the every-day visual field, for they are very much more beautiful than anything we ever see when we have not taken mescaline.

Hallucinatory sense-experience is delusive in the sense that it gives us no reliable information about the biologically important physical world, but it does give us information about the aesthetically interesting hallucinatory world. Therefore it is better to call Ayer's 'veridical' sense-experience *ordinary* sense-experience, and refrain from calling hallucinatory sense-experience *delusive*, or, if we do, we must qualify our statement by calling it *biologically delusive*.

12.3. In any event it is not of fundamental epistemological importance whether we call hallucinatory sense-experience real or unreal. To ask if an hallucination is real or unreal is to ask what are the criteria which we have laid down to govern the use of the word ⟨real⟩ in our epistemological system. But to ask if an hallucination is spatial or if it is coloured is to ask questions which can be answered by direct observation. A man can only bear witness to the nature of his own hallucinations and the hallucinations I noticed on the two occasions that I took mescaline seemed to be best to merit the description of spatial (and coloured) entities. They certainly exhibited an internal spatial organisation as well as belonging to an external spatial system in that they bore spatial relations to other sense-data.

Thus we must modify Ayer's criteria to say that we can distinguish between hallucinatory and ordinary sense-experience by noting the *particular* order to which any given sense-experience or series of sense-experiences belongs and by noting the *particular* type of predictions that further sense-experiences will confirm. Which of these two orders we choose to call *real* depends very much upon the orientation of our particular culture into which we have been born, and in the midst of which we have grown up, to bear its stamp upon the whole system of our thought. People vary very greatly in their attitude towards hallucinatory sense-experience. This attitude is largely determined by cultural factors. In our culture an hallucinatory experience is usually something shameful. People who have them usually keep quiet about them for fear that they be considered mad. People in other cultures attach very great importance to hallucinatory experiences. For instance, it was the belief of the Plains Indians that a man's success in life was obtained in a dream or vision.

'On the western plains men sought these visions with hideous tortures. They cut strips from the skin of their arms, they struck off fingers, they swung themselves from tall poles by straps inserted under the muscles of their shoulders. They went without food or water for extreme periods. They sought in every way to achieve an order of experience set apart from daily living.'[1]

Western people in the early Christian era pursued hallucinatory experiences with an equally passionate intensity believing them to provide a direct method of communication with the supernatural world. The hallucinatory world to these people was at least as real as the ordinary world. The traditional Hindu culture, on the other hand, regarded neither orders of experience to be real. They classed ordinary and hallucinatory experience together as 'maya' or illusion. The term 'real' was reserved for the immanent Godhead. This highly sophisticated philosophy regarded the hallucinatory visions, so prized by Catholic mystics and by the Indians of the American plains, and 'veridical' sense-experience, which is the only form of experience recognised as *real* by our culture, as equally illusory and serving only to distract man from his proper goal—union with the Godhead. Thus the decision to call only ordinary sense-experi-

[1] Ruth Benedict, *Patterns of Culture* (Mentor Book edition), p. 74.

ence real is a local phenomenon of Western European culture. It is also contingent upon the biochemical accident that our adrenal glands happen to produce adrenaline and not adrenochrome or mescaline. A valid philosophical criteria of the real should not be contingent upon cultural factors and biochemical accidents.

12.4. This consideration of the empirical facts of hallucinatory sense-experience allows us to make the following statements.

12.41. Sense-experience exhibits two great systems of order: that is to say it can be classified significantly in the following ways. In one the sense-data are so ordered as to represent as constantly as possible parts of the physical world. In the other, sense-data are ordered so as to construct patterns, designs, scenes and panoramic vistas of the greatest possible beauty, poetical integrity and aesthetic charm.

12.42. All sensory experiences are equally real. Any sense-experience will belong to a greater or lesser extent to one or other of these two orders. In fact, we can choose, if we so wish, to lay down our criteria of reality (without going outside the limits of Ayer's generalised criteria) to ensure that the *type of order* and the *type of predictions* will usually be satisfied by certain types of hallucinatory sense-experience and not by 'veridical' experiences. It will be admitted that our criteria will not be biologically useful but they will have, in a Pickwickian sense, aesthetic merit.

12.5. Hallucinations also pose a physiological problem. For the usual physiological explanation for them is to say that they are the same patterns of neuronal stimulation in the cortex as are normally aroused by seeing physical objects, evoked in the case of hallucinatory sense-experience in the absence of such external objects and thus without the usual activity in the sub-cortical perceptual apparatus. But it is clear, for the neuroanatomical reasons already given, that sense-data, ordinary or hallucinatory, cannot be identical with any patterns of neuronal excitation in the brain. If they cannot *be* these patterns the problem arises of what sort of entities they are and how they are related to these brain patterns, to which, in some cases, they are certainly causally related, as in those cases where hallucinatory sense-experiences are evoked by electrical stimulation of the brain. These are not problems for the representative Theories I and II, as sense-data, in these theories, are spatial parts of the mind and are not in the same place as the neuronal patterns of excitation in the brain.

We can postulate, therefore, that the mescaline phenomena are the autonomous activity of the sensory fields. That is to say, we can suggest that the afferent causal relations between the brain and the sensory fields are not wholly *excitatory* (as in normal vision), but that they are *inhibitory* as well. Thus mescaline may be supposed to inhibit that function of the brain which specifically inhibits the mescaline phenomena from developing in the sensory fields. Now, if the self (the 'observer', Pure Ego, witness, etc.: see 13.3) survives the dissolution of the physical body, as it may do if Theories I or II are true statements, then it clearly cannot continue to have what we now call veridical sense experiences. But if the hypothesis given above is correct (i.e. that the brain actively *inhibits* certain activities of the mind), then the Self may witness the 'mescaline' phenomena in the degree to which these may develop following their total release from the inhibitory function of the brain. Now mescaline certainly inhibits the oxidative mechanisms of the brain (although probably through an intermediary mechanism) but, of course, it is also possible that the mescaline phenomena are not the autonomous activity of the visual field: they may be generated wholly by the disordered brain mechanisms via the usual excitatory causal relations (i.e. ψ_y) between the brain and mind. Both hypotheses are logically possible. It is also possible that the Self may not survive the destruction of the physical body even if Theories I or II are true statements.

12.6. One way in which we might maintain the current scientific assumption that the Universe consists of only one four-dimensional spatio-temporal system might be as follows: It could be asserted that the only existent spatial entities were physical objects which we would experience directly. It would then be stated that there were no such spatial entities as images or hallucinations but only *processes* of imaging and hallucinating. Ryle[1] has argued in this manner with respect to imaging.

---

[1] Gilbert Ryle (a), *The Concept of Mind*, London, 1949.

Thus, it would be alleged, it would not make sense to talk of spatial relations between 'hallucinatory sense-data' and physical objects because there would not be any such entities as hallucinations or hallucinatory sense-data. Similarly one could not say that images bore spatial relations to anything any more than one could say that there were spatial relations between an orange and a guess or the process of guessing.

However, it is certain[d] that hallucinations are themselves spatially extended, their parts bearing spatial relations to each other; and hallucinatory sense-data bear spatial relations to other hallucinatory sense-data and to veridical sense-data. This can be put as follows. We must accept that in normal perception we are immediately aware of spatial objects (it does not matter for the purpose of this argument whether we call these objects *physical objects* or *sense-data* or 'complete optical objects' in Broad's sense or 'sensible-objects' in Woodger's sense). It cannot be denied that hallucinations of class (ii) bear direct (sensible) spatial relations to the objects in the veridical remainder of the visual field. Only spatial entities can bear spatial relations to other spatial entities. Therefore hallucinations are spatial entities.

In any case, from the point of view of Theories I and II, all that it is necessary to establish is that the statements 'sense-data (in this case hallucinatory sense-data) can bear spatial relations to physical objects' and 'sense-data can form a spatial system outside that of the physical world' are meaningful statements. If one now holds that we experience external physical objects directly in visual perception we can say that hallucinations do bear spatial relations to these objects. Then, if we reject naïve realism, there is nothing to prevent sense-data from bearing spatial relations of another kind to physical objects or from forming, together with other sense-data and images, a spatial system different from that of the physical world. The empirical facts forbid us, however, from postulating that (1) any ordinary sense-data, or (2) hallucinatory sense-data or (3) images could ever form a spatial system in which the other two were not included for the spatial relations between (1), (2) and (3) may be confirmed by direct observation.

A similar type of argument may be used against Ryle's

contention that there are no such entities as images but only processes of imaging. For parts of an image bear spatial relations to other parts of the same image and to other images. A guess does not bear spatial relations to other guesses.

Furthermore people who have hallucinatory experiences very often do describe them in the same terms as they use to describe what they see when they are not having hallucinations. They said 'I see', 'as I gazed', 'It is wonderful to see', etc. A study of the examples given in 12.1 shows that only once did one of the observers say in a perceptual statement 'I seemed [to be gazing]'. On the three occasions on which he uses the word 'seem' Weir Mitchell is not making perceptual statements but is using ⟨seem⟩ in its poetical descriptive sense. To say 'all seemed to be possessed of an interior light' is equivalent to saying 'the mountains seem quite ethereal in the spring' or 'this speech seems to be largely hogwash'. In Weir Mitchell's perceptual statements he says 'as I gazed', 'as I looked', 'I saw', and not 'as I seemed to gaze', 'as I seemed to look', 'as I seemed to see'. Similarly Knauer or Maloney says 'above me *is* a dome' etc. The language that they use indicates that they consider themselves to be confronted with an objective reality quite apart from them distinct from their own personality or organism—that there are merely a lot of things going on out there which they can observe and report on. The experience has a great deal in common with ordinary sense-perception and it has something, but much less, in common with imaging (occasionally what is seen can be influenced directly by the subject).

12.7. In his most recent work Ryle[1] presents a defence of the common-sense belief that we do gain true knowledge about the world by means of our sense-experience. He argues against the following propositions put forward by some philosophers, (12.71) because some of our perceptions are illusory or hallucinatory, therefore all our knowledge about the external world is suspect; and (12.72) that in perception we really perceive events going on in our own brains or in our own minds.

The physiologist can reply to Ryle's arguments as follows:

12.73. It is possible to give a physiological account of percep-

---

[1] Gilbert Ryle (*b*), *Dilemmas*, Cambridge, 1954.

tion which uses the words ⟨see⟩, ⟨look at⟩, ⟨regard⟩, etc., so as not to challenge the validity of common-sense statements of the form 'I see a cow', 'I am looking at a beetle', etc. No physiologist need ever say[1] 'Observers, including the physiologists and psychologists themselves, never perceive what they naïvely suppose themselves to perceive', or again,[2] 'From some well-known facts of optics, acoustics and physiology it seemed to follow that what we see, hear or smell cannot be, as we ordinarily suppose, things and happenings outside us, but are on the contrary, things and happenings inside us.' The facts of physiology, neurology, and experimental psychology indicate, not that our common-sense knowledge about the external physical world is suspect, but that we are mistaken in our common-sense beliefs about how the physiological processes, that mediate our perception of objects, function. That is to say that statements of the kind 'There is a typewriter in the room' or 'That cow is red' may be true or false according to the circumstances, but statements of the kind 'We look at the world through our senses or through our eyes' or 'He glanced out of the corner of his eyes' are false. Linguistic philosophers would do well to consider to what extent statements about perception in common usage ('correct' English) reflect folk (and erroneous) beliefs about the manner in which the perceptual apparatus functions. Such phrases as '*through* the senses' and ' I glanced *out of* the corner of my eye' suggest that we look out at the world through (or out of) our eyes as we look out of a window at the scene outside (i.e. that the visual perceptual apparatus works like a simple optical instrument which is a folk belief incompatible with neurological knowledge). The physiologist's account would run as follows: Perceiving (regarding, looking at) a physical object is nothing but the physiological (and physical) process: physical object—light—retina—brain—sense-datum, together with the sensing of the latter. The empirical evidence presented above suggests that the sense-data we are aware of in our direct experience are not parts of, nor are they, the physical objects themselves. The physiologist can use the technical term *sensing* to describe his present relation to his own sense-data. Thus he can say that the physiological processes of perception

[1] Ryle, loc. cit. (*b*), p. 94.   [2] *Ibid.*, p. 109.

99

mediate our perception of the external world, and an essential *part* of this process is the sensing of sense-data constructed by these physiological processes. The relation between perceiving and sensing is thus that of whole to part. Thus, as was demonstrated above, we do perceive what we naïvely suppose we perceive. But we do not sense the same objects that we perceive. There is no warrant in any of this to suggest that the physiologist's account of perception brings into doubt any of our common-sense knowledge about the world.[1] This whole problem was extensively analysed in Chapter 1.

12.74. Ryle bases his argument (that, even if some of our perceptions do turn out to be illusory or hallucinatory, we cannot then claim that all our perceptions may be illusory or hallucinatory, and so we have no need to entertain a chronic state of doubt about the validity of all our knowledge about ordinary things) on the grounds that the existence of fakes logically presupposes the existence of some genuine articles, of which we can have fakes or counterfeits. 'For there must be an answer to the question "counterfeits of what" '. But what justification have we for supposing that sensory illusions and hallucinations are fakes or counterfeits of real perceptions or things? To be a counterfeit or a fake an object must, so common usage has it, have been constructed by a man, or found in nature by a man, and then used with the psychological intention of personal gain (of any kind) through fraud. If an event is a fake (e.g. a fake funeral) it must be executed by a person or group of people with the intent to defraud or possibly entertain. Hallucinations and illusions are merely certain types of experience different from the general order of our experience (or rather, as all our sensory experience contains an illusory element—a constant-size effect or some distortion of visual objects in the peripheral visual field for example—they are different from some ideal illusionless sensory experience never realised: they are only different in degree from our ordinary sense experience) and cannot be called false, counterfeit or faked. *Actions* arising out of an hallucinatory

[1] Thus it will be noted that this account differs from the traditional Lockean account in that it is not claimed that 'what is externally real is never perceived', but merely that we do not sense the same entities that we perceive.

sense-experience may not be relevant to the environmental situation (and the criteria as to what is relevant behaviour in response to an hallucinatory sense-experience are culturally determined: compare our reactions to those of the Plains Indians described above). Similarly *beliefs* aroused by an hallucinatory sense-experience may be false if a belief proper to one order of experience is illegitimately transferred to the other; we can have true and false beliefs, as we can have knowledge, about hallucinations (e.g. that some hallucinations are coloured). Thus I would also reject the views of those philosophers that Ryle is attacking with his argument but for different reasons. Their mistake has been to suppose that, because some hallucinatory experiences have lead to erroneous judgments and false beliefs on or about events in the physical world, that this gives us grounds to doubt *all* judgments and beliefs on or about events in the physical world. We can deny these grounds, not for the reason that hallucinations are some kind of counterfeit veridical experience, but for the reason that veridical sense-experiences satisfy our ordinary criteria by which we judge what are true statements about external events and what are false, whereas hallucinatory sense-experiences do not satisfy these criteria. Note however that statements about hallucinations can also be true.

12.75. Ryle's second main argument in this chapter is that it is futile to attempt to give a physiological account of what goes on in perception in terms of *process* because, as he argues, the verb ⟨see⟩ is not usually used[1] to signify an experience gone through or engaged in, nor does it signify a process because it belongs to a family of verbs like ⟨find⟩, ⟨detect⟩, and ⟨solve⟩, —verbs of starting and stopping—which do not stand for[2] 'processes taking place in or to things, or for states in which things remain.' He contrasts the verb ⟨see⟩ with the verb ⟨look⟩ which does stand for a temporal process with a start, middle and end—'I looked at the picture for ten seconds.' Thus a defence against Ryle's argument presents itself. The physiologist can correlate his account not with seeing but with looking or watching or peering or gazing, which are just as much

[1] But it may so be used, e.g. 'I saw him as clearly as I *am seeing* you now.'
[2] Ryle, loc. cit. (*b*), p. 104.

modes of visual perception under certain conditions as is seeing. It must be noted that Ryle makes an illegitimate step in his argument. Even if he has made his point about ⟨seeing⟩ (see note 1 over) he claims to have shown that it is not true that[1] *'perceiving* is a bodily process or state, as perspiring is; or that it is a non-bodily or psychological process or state; or, perhaps, that it is somehow jointly a bodily and a non-bodily process or state'. [My italics.] Note the illegitimate substitution of ⟨perceiving⟩ for ⟨seeing⟩. He has made out his case for ⟨seeing⟩ and not for ⟨perceiving⟩. His whole argument breaks down for ⟨looking⟩. Yet *looking* is as much a mode of visual perception as is *seeing*. In any case we can directly observe the physiological processes of perception at work in the stroboscopic phenomena.

12.8. THE LOGICAL ANALYSIS OF LANGUAGE AS A MEANS OF STUDYING PERCEPTION

The 'logical analysis of language' approach to perception proceeds by studying statements made about perception. One way of doing this is to study statements made about sense-data and statements made about physical objects and searching for logical relations between these statements. It might then approach the problems discussed in this chapter as follows. It would consider the two statements 'sense-data are spatial entities' (or 1a 'sense-data bear spatial relations to other sense-data') and 2 'physical objects are spatial entities' (or 2a 'physical objects bear spatial relations to other physical objects'). It might then try to relate these statements logically. Could this method be used to prove logically that the statements 3 'sense-data bear spatial relations to physical objects' and 3a 'sense-data do not bear spatial relations to physical objects' are meaningless? It could only attempt to do so by making the sole criteria of meaning the 'standards of correctness in English'. In this case the only reason for calling these statements 'meaningless' would be because ordinary people do not use technical terms like sense-data in their everyday conversation, and thus we could not find such statements in their conversation. But we cannot

[1] Ryle, oc. cit. (*b*), p. 109.

accept these criteria of meaning in the case of technical terms like ⟨sense-data⟩.

12.81. We may further doubt if the philosophical method of linguistic analysis is altogether a sound one if carried to excess. To base one's study of perception or one's criticism of comprehensive physiological and neurological theories of perception on an analysis of the grammatical structure of the English language and on what are called 'the standards of correct English usage' is to overlook the following point. The basic form of our language depends on two factors: (1) this basic form was constructed by our remote ancestors and (2) its continued use depends on the uncritical acceptance of these patterns of language by each generation. The patterns themselves are transmitted wholly by learning as are any other patterns of culture. As Whorf puts it:[1]

'Natural logic contains two fallacies: First, it does not see that the phenomena of a language are to its own speakers largely of a background character and so are outside the critical consciousness and control of the speaker who is expounding natural logic. Hence, when anyone, as a natural logician, is talking about reason, logic, and the laws of correct thinking, he is apt to be simply marching in step with purely grammatical facts that have somewhat of a background character in his own language or family of languages but are by no means universal in all languages and in no sense a common substratum of reason. Second, natural logic confuses agreement about subject matter, attained through use of language, with knowledge of the linguistic process by which agreement is attained, . . .

'The categories and types that we isolate from the world of phenomena we do not find there because they stare every observer in the face; on the contrary, the world is presented in a kaleidoscopic flux of impressions which has to be organised by our minds—and this means largely by the linguistic systems in our minds. We cut nature up, organise it into concepts, and ascribe significances as we do, largely because we are parties to an agreement to organise it in this way—an agreement that holds throughout our speech community and is codified in the patterns of our language. The agreement is, of course, an im-

[1] B. L. Whorf, *Four Articles on Metalinguistics*, Foreign Service Institute, Department of State, Washington, 1950, pp. 4–5.

plicit and unstated one, *but its terms are absolutely obligatory*; we cannot talk at all except by subscribing to the organisation and classification of data which the agreement decrees.'

Thus, when linguistic philosophers attempt to answer philosophical questions by studying what they call the logical basis of language, part of what they will be studying will be 'natural logic'—this implicit and unstated agreement codified in the patterns of our language. To some extent this agreement is based on arbitrary and illogical (or better alogical) criteria. These are not the sort of criteria recognised by formal logic. Whorf gives as an example the way in which we decide whether a given natural feature is a *thing* or an *event* and shows that an analysis of such major structural features of a language, as we might undertake in answer to the question 'what do nouns and verbs stand for?' will give somewhat different results as we study different languages. Similarly a study of the classification of verbs of perception may give different results in different languages. If we construct any philosophy, or a theory of perception, on a basis of the grammatical forms found in English, together with an analysis of the finest nuances to be gleaned from ordinary conversation, we might have to construct a different account of perception if we study the Hopi language, another if we study Nootka, another if we study an Eskimo language, etc. We cannot merely make the ethnocentric assumption that *English*, or Standard Average European, hold the key to all philosophical dilemmas. As Whorf says:[1]

'But to restrict thinking to the patterns merely of English, and especially to those patterns which represent the acme of plainness in English, is to lose a power of thought which, once lost, can never be regained. It is the "plainest" English which contains the greatest number of unconscious assumptions about nature. . . . Western culture has made, through language, a provisional analysis of reality and, without correctives, holds resolutely to that analysis as final. The only correctives lie in all those other tongues which by aeons of independent evolution have arrived at different, but equally logical, provisional analyses.'"

[1] Whorf, loc. cit., pp. 22–3.

Veridical and Hallucinatory Sense-Experience

In particular, anthropologists have made it plain that an important determining factor in the development of science has been the necessity for questioning some item in this implicit agreement and for escaping from the clichés of our language. Thus it is not a valid criticism of any scientific account of perception to show that it does not conform in some particular feature with common usage or the 'standards of correctness in English'. For the physiologist has only to reply that the standards of correctness in common English usage represent only one of a number of possible and equally valid ways of analysing experience. The standards of correctness have been subject to modification, introduced into the language by influential philosophers and scientists in the past. The physiologist is perfectly justified in using technical terms such as 'sense-data' or 'sensing' and for giving accounts of the way that the perceptual apparatus may function that conflict with the account given by common usage, if he can show good empirical reasons for doing so. If his analysis obtains general agreement amongst other scientists and philosophers, and particularly if he can make predictions that may be confirmed by experiment, then his terms and his account of perception will pass first into general scientific usage, and later into general lay usage, and once again the 'standards of correctness in English' will be changed in conformity with that which science has been able to discover about nature—in this instance, about the natural processes of perception.

Chapter Five

EXAMINATION OF 'PERCEPTION¹'

<hr/>

13.   IT is my purpose in this chapter to examine Price's theory of perception. I will attempt to establish that he has made two unwitting primary assumptions, which may well be erroneous, and that the presence of these assumptions gives rise to a certain confusion in his argument, and leads him to make erroneous conclusions as to the nature of sense-data and their relation to physical objects.

13.1   THE STANDARD SOLID AND PHYSICAL OBJECTS

The first questions that may be raised concern the nature of Price's *physical object* and *standard solid*:

(*a*) Is the physical object literally extended in space?

(*b*) Does the standard solid, as defined, literally make up a three-dimensional solid?

(*c*) What is the nature of the relation of 'coincidence' that he says exists between physical objects and standard solids?

To start with (*a*): It is difficult to make out if Price believes that physical objects are literally extended in space or not. He starts off by saying:

'But can we say anything more about physical objects except that they possess such and such causal characteristics (impenetrability or obstacularity being in every case one of them)? We

¹ 2nd Edition, revised 1950.

106

can say that they have such and such sizes, shapes and positions at such and such dates, and that they change these in various ways' (p. 294).

He goes on to suggest that we can infer that physical objects have *intrinsic qualities* of some kind or other:

'For nothing can have only causal characteristics, . . . it follows from the very nature of relations that the whole being of something cannot consist in its relations to other things—else there would be nothing to be related' (p. 294).

But it turns out to be impossible to state exactly what these intrinsic qualities are. Size and position are relational qualities and 'shape cannot constitute the intrinsic nature of anything—else there would be nothing to be "shaped" ' (p. 294). He mentions Broad's suggestion that—'some at least one of these intrinsic qualities must be "spread out" or "extensible" in the way in which colour is spread out over a visual sense-datum'; but he decides that this really does not follow from what we know although it may still be true. 'Physical occupation', Price continues, 'is of a purely *causal* sort' (p. 295), and he gives as an analogy the military and legal sorts of occupation. He says later:

'a physical occupant of the ordinary macroscopic sort is *defined* as a causally characterised entity with which a family of sense-data is coincident' (p. 302); and again: 'But a pure physical object is something so shadowy that we can scarcely conceive of it at all' (p. 303).

The following statements are crucial:

'Of course, a physical object may also sometimes or always occupy a place in some further way, which does resemble sensory occupation; but we have no positive reason for thinking that it does' (p. 295); 'we do not know the intrinsic characteristics upon which physical, i.e., *space-occupational*, characteristics are dependent' (p. 297—my italics).

It is difficult to make out from this account if physical objects are extended in space or not. The verdict seems to be that we do not know and have no way of knowing but they may well be. Yet in the last quotation given above 'physical' is identified with 'space-occupational'.

Now the nature of the relationship of 'coincidence', which is frequently given as holding between standard solids and physical objects, surely depends on this question as to whether physical objects are extended in space or not? Even if we do not know the answer to this question it is possible to distinguish between the implications inherent in the two possible answers. For instance, if physical objects are extended in space ('spread out' or 'extensible'), then the relationship of coincidence becomes *geometrical*, and the first assumption that Price has made at once becomes obvious. He has merely assumed that this relationship would be one of *geometrical coincidence*, whereas it is possible to formulate alternative geometrical relations (see Chapter 1). But, if physical objects are not so extended, this relationship of 'coincidence' means something else. Here all the spatial qualities of material things derive from their standard solid components, and in this region certain causal characteristics manifest themselves. Thus there are not two geometrical entities to be related and the question of what may be the actual geometrical relationship between them does not arise. Surely, however, it seems more probable that physical objects such as the earth and the stars possess the intrinsic quality of extension in space rather than that they do not? And if they are so extended the question of the actual geometrical relation between physical subjects and sensa or standard solids may have to be dealt with.

This issue also arises in Price's definition of physical space. If physical objects are extended in space, then physical space is the space system in which they are extended. But Price defines physical space thus:

'Finally, we may ask whether visual and tactual sense-data have positions in what some would wish us to call "the Space of Standard Solids". (This is the same as "physical" or "public" space)' (p. 246).

Thus it is assumed that physical space is that in which *standard solids* are extended. If physical objects are not extended in space, then it is clear that material things and standard solids are extended in the same 'physical' space, since the standard solid is the only spatial component of the material thing. But if physical objects are themselves spatial entities (and not merely shadowy *nexūs* of causal characteristics), then this is not at all obvious, since the actual spatial extension of material things may derive from their physical object component, and not from their standard solid component, if the space of physical objects does not happen to be coincident with the space of standard solids.

We must now deal with the process of derivation of the standard solid. He describes the set of nuclear sense-data making up the standard solid thus; '. . . all the members of it at any one moment fit together to form a single three-dimensional whole' (p. 276). If we go through the actions Price prescribes whereby such a standard solid is constructed, we find that no such actual solid can be constructed out of sensa or any groups of them. However much and for however long we manipulate objects, or walk round them, while the sense-data belonging to them shrink and grow and change their shapes and relative positions, we are always dealing with a unitary visual field and no such complete three-dimensional solid object can ever be conjured out of this field in time. Price recognises this himself when he calls the process not one of construction but of syngnosis (p. 310). Thus the process of 'progressive adjunction' described by Price, gives us not a complete three-dimensional standard solid constructed out of sense-data, but it merely confirms our knowledge (conscious or unconscious, naïve or sophisticated) that *material* things themselves (and not standard solids) are complete three-dimensional solids. When we analyse Price's method of progressive adjunction, we find that in the crucial second paragraph on page 227, where the distortion series and the differentiation series are united into one system, we turn suddenly away from an examination of pure sense-data and visual *imagery* is brought into play:

'All we have now to do is to take the most differentiated member of the series and, as it were, *conflate it in imagination* with the nuclear datum which is its limit. That is, *we must imagine it* keeping all its differentiatedness and losing its distortion, or *we may imagine* the nuclear datum keeping its constructibility and losing its relatively undifferentiated character; the two alternatives come *as far as shape goes* to exactly the same thing' (p. 227 —my italics).

Thus, at this crucial moment in the construction of the standard solid in Price's mind, he suddenly leaves the actual sense-data themselves and proceeds to exercise his own imagery, which it must be remembered has its own spatial nature. Ayer does much the same thing:[1]

'And by this means one can provide oneself also with a set of sense-data which can be fitted together in the imagination, like the pieces of a jigsaw puzzle, in such a way as to yield a complete picture of the object, which may never as a whole be given to sense.'

It is however evident that, whereas we can fit *images* together in our imaginations 'like the pieces of a jigsaw puzzle', we cannot so fit *sense-data*. Thus the standard solid is in actuality an hybrid of sensa and imagery, and even with this admixture of imagery it does not make up a complete closed three-dimensional solid. There seems to be somewhat of a strain about this whole business of the standard solids. There is a feeling that they are being called upon to do more than they can actually do. When we investigate this we find that they are being forced to be actual, three-dimensional solids to make up the spatial component of material things. For if we are convinced that they do so, then we do not have to raise the question as to whether this role may not in fact be played by the physical object component, which leads in turn to the question as to what may be the spatial relation between physical objects and the various sensory fields. In fact we may even doubt whether standard solids play any part in the actual construction of material objects.

All visual sensa, nuclear and non-nuclear, have their primary positions in the spatial system of their visual fields—they always possess sensible spatial relations to other sense-data within the visual field during the same specious present. Any theory that seeks to put groups of nuclear sense-data in one 'space' and all other sense-data in some other 'space' is invalid. For it would entail that nuclear sense-data could not bear any sensible spatial relations to other sense-data within the same visual field during the same specious present. It is, however, an empirical fact that any sense-datum within the visual field during any specious present bears spatial relations to all other sense-data within the

[1] Ayer, loc. cit., p. 250.

same visual field during the same specious present. The standard solid is a semi-abstract hybrid of sensa and imagery: that which has spatial location at any time is always merely the sense-datum or collection of sense-data in the unitary visual field.

The argument that Price uses to get round this on pages 250–2, in which he says that the relation of a nuclear sense-datum to a standard solid is not a spatial one but is one of being a constituent of it and 'the manner of constituting is given by progressive adjunction' is most ingenious. Nuclear data are thus not in the space of standard solids but bear a more fundamental relation to them, that of 'being a constituent of'. But this does not really get round the problem, for the spatial relation to the group of standard solids is now possessed by a 'certain group of sense-data . . . and [by] nothing less'. The sense-data composing these groups still bear very definite spatial relations in their own visual fields during any one specious present. These spatial relations are always quite clear and primary and form one single and unitary spatial system. We must then relate the members of these groups of nuclear sense-data, which are alleged to be constituents of the standard solids, to *all the other sense-data making up the total visual field throughout the same specious present.* The nuclear and non-nuclear sense-data belonging to any one object both bear these latter relations, and it is *these* relations that prevent nuclear sense-data from being in one 'space' and non-nuclear ones in another. In concentrating upon one optical object Price neglects the rest of the visual field, which is illegitimate since the visual field is always a unitary whole, which fact is the basis of Gestalt psychology.

If I take a book in my hand and move it about to obtain the nuclear data, and if I walk round it to obtain the same, it is quite certain that all the sense-data obtained belong to a single continuous four-dimensional manifold (the total visual field in time) of which they form parts and that no combination of them can form an actual complete three-dimensional solid during any one specious present.[1] The following arguments seem to establish

[1] Even if I close my eyes during this process the manifold is not disturbed. The complex visual field containing the book turns momentarily into a single black or reddish datum filling the whole field in which the after-image of the book and surroundings rapidly fades.

this. If I look at the front of an object and obtain the nuclear sense-datum for that, will not the nuclear datum for the back, which I obtained two minutes before, have actually to be there now almost back to back with the front datum—separated by the thickness of the object—to make up the single three-dimensional standard solid? Furthermore with this datum for the back will there not have to be the rest of the visual field in which it was embedded and with which it formed one single organic whole—literally there and now? Again how does one obtain the standard solid for an *irregular* object such as a knobby stone? Any view of such an object will always contain nuclear and non-nuclear data hopelessly intermingled. Price avoids this point by only considering regular objects such as match boxes. The standard solid as defined is never a complete three-dimensional solid but is a curious four-dimensional *open* entity. It is more like a projection of this solid on to the complex surface of the visual field.

If extension in space be attributed to the physical object, then there is no need to invent such an entity as the standard solid. Visual sense-data may be allowed to have their actually sensed extended shapes and spatial relations embedded in their own unitary sense-fields. The three-dimensional solidity that we all feel material things do have may derive from the physical object, which may even make up the whole of the material thing. This is certainly simpler than the standard solid theory. The whole question may then be reduced to a consideration of the possible geometrical relationships between sense-data and physical objects.

13.2. THE SOMATIC SENSORY FIELD AND THE PHYSICAL BODY

The second point to be raised concerns the relation between the somatic datum (or the somatic sensory field—s.s.f. for short —in which I include touch, pain, temperature, and all types of pressure and proprioceptive sense-data) and the physical organism. At times in this book Price assumes that the s.s.f. is in fact coincident with the physical body. For instance, in the argument on pages 39–41 seeking to relate sense-data with the brain or physical organism, the relations given actually hold between visual sense-data (or v.s.d.) and somatic sense-data (or s.s.d.). For instance, on pages 38–9, he says that because 'somatic and environmental sense-data are always co-present and co-variant' it does not necessarily follow that 'all sense-data are products of the brain'. But he then goes on to discuss the relations between environmental and somatic sense-data as though the latter necessarily *contained* the brain. But this is clearly a mistake. The relevant relationship is v.s.d. *plus* s.s.d. (= Price's Total Datum) to the physical organism. The fact that v.s.d. are never found apart from s.s.d. tells us nothing about the relation of both these to the physical organism, and to suppose that s.s.d. are instrumental in enabling us to sense environmental data is not the same as supposing that the physical organism (of which the brain is a structural part) does this. If physiological idealism states that s.s.d. create environmental data, physiological realism would state that the organism creates both somatic and environmental data.

Physiological Idealism: s.s.d. $\rightarrow$ v.s.d.
Physiological Realism: Physical organism $\rightarrow$ s.s.d.
                                                                   $\searrow$ v.s.d.

Similarly in the arguments developed on pages 127–31 Price clearly locates the physical brain inside the sensed skull. It is certain that v.s.d. are outside the sensed skull but this is only to say that they are outside the s.s.f. It cannot be taken for granted that the sensed skull *is* the physical skull or is coincident with it in any way. *If* v.s.d. are to be cerebral events then so must be s.s.d., and both sets of sense-data must literally be inside the physical brain inside the physical skull.

Similarly on page 134 the two series of events 'separated by a blank interval of "outness" ' are visual sense-data and somatic sense-data and not v.s.d. and the physical organism. *One cannot relate v.s.d. to s.s.d. in the belief that one is necessarily relating sense-data in general to the physical organism.* Since Price does just this his arguments about the cerebral or psychical status of sense-data break down. He summarises these arguments thus:

'in various ways the relation of sense-data to events which

admittedly inhere in the brain and the self is not at all the same as the relation of those events to one another' (p. 134).

Now:

(i) In the spatial way, the somatic sensory field is identified with the physical organism on the validity of which identification it is possible to cast much doubt.

(ii) In the way of discontinuity in respect of quality, Price neglects the existence of experiences of synaesthesia which certainly do fill in this gap.

(iii) In respect of sequence his argument would still hold even if sense-data were cerebral events, since they would only be a small portion of the total cerebral activity. Events in other parts of the brain would help to determine the total state of the brain and thus the behaviour of the person, which could not then in any case be inferable directly from a mere inspection of sense-data.

There certainly are other reasons against sense-data being located in the brain which we have already reviewed in Chapter I. The most important is that they are geometrically entirely *incongruent* with any possible patterns of neuronal excitation in the brain. There is nothing however to prevent them from being parts of the mind, *if* this is then regarded as being spatially extended and organised in its own right.

Broad also assumes that the s.s.f. is identical with the physical organisation.[1]

'There is one and only one literal sense of "being in a place". This is not definable, but it is exemplified in our sense-experience most clearly in the presence of a visual sensum at a certain sensible place in its visual field. The concept of being in a place is based on our sensible acquaintance with such instances as this. It can then be applied in thought to types of object and of continuum which we cannot sense as simultaneous wholes. Again, there is one and one only kind of place which we deal with when once we *leave individual sensa and their fields and pass to physical objects* in the widest sense of the term. This is a place in the continuum of possible positions of *our bodies* as we move. This continuum is not sensed as a simultaneous whole; but our successive experiences of motion are synthesised under the con-

---

[1] Broad, loc. cit. (*b*), p. 333—my italics.

cept of a spatial whole, through analogy with visual fields which we can sense simultaneously.'

If we examine some visual sense-data and then turn our attention to the somatic sense-data making up the sensed body we are not necessarily leaving a sense-field and passing to a physical object. Furthermore it does not seem that we can sense the somatic sensory field as any less of a spatial whole than we can the visual field. If, when we cease to attend to a visual sense-datum and turn our attention to a somatic sense-datum, this is taken necessarily to imply that the s.s.f. is literally identical with the physical body, then we have already committed ourselves to a relation between sense-data and physical objects from which we will never be able to escape again. The s.s.f. at any one moment is a spatial whole (and surely for blind people it is the only spatial whole), and the concept of a spatial whole upon which we base our concept of physical space is derived as much from our experience of the somatic sensory field as it is from the visual field. In congenitally blind people the s.s.f. is the only source of spatial concepts, which, although different from the spatial concepts of the sighted, are nevertheless spatial concepts. Thus, while the *concept* of the movement continuum is based on our experience of the spatio-temporal system of the s.s.f., it cannot be taken for granted that the physical body and the s.s.f. are identical.

13.3. THE USE OF THE WORDS ⟨SELF⟩, ⟨MIND⟩ AND ⟨CONSCIOUSNESS⟩

Price uses the word ⟨mind⟩ in many places to denote the Self or Witness. If the latter is called *mind* there is surely a danger of prejudicing the issue with respect to the status, mental or otherwise, of the sensa of which the Witness is aware? Since the words like ⟨Ego⟩ and ⟨Self⟩ have different meanings according to who uses them (cf. the Freudian's use of ⟨Ego⟩) I suggest that the fine old word ⟨Witness⟩[1] should be used to denote the

[1] It does not matter for the purposes of this argument whether the Witness be thought of as a continuant entity (the Vedantist view) or as a series of acts of awareness (the Buddhist view).

essential experiencing being who is *aware* of, or senses, the sense and imagery fields presented to him, or to his awareness. The whole system of Witness,[1] sense and images, thoughts and feelings, would then make up the totality of *consciousness* or the conscious mind. Thus the simplest ordinary perceptual situation would be then a Witness is sensing or is aware of a particular sensum embedded in its field of surrounding sensa. In this case there is no related activity going on in the thought or imagery fields.[2] If, however, we name the object or recognise it the proper symbol arises in the thought field. More complex types of 'apprehending that' (p. 5) arise from more complex process occurring in the thought field. The processes of genesis of the visual field and the sensing of the data so generated on the one hand and the selection and presentation of the proper symbols on the other, demonstrably depend on different cerebral processes. The latter process may be disturbed or even abolished by a cerebral lesion giving rise to *agnosia* without any gross effect on the former process. The processes of genesis of the visual field may similarly be disturbed in many complex ways (giving rise to spatial disorganisation of the visual field, macropsia, micropsia, metamorphopsia, hemianopsia, apparent movement, space colours, etc.) without any effect on the other (see Chapter 2).

Now Price uses ⟨mind⟩ in many places where I would use ⟨Witness⟩, e.g. on pages 11, 21, 22, 31, 93, 285, and 296. He also uses ⟨consciousness⟩ where I would use ⟨awareness⟩, e.g. 'this whole field of colour is directly present to my consciousness' (p. 3). Would it not be better to say 'present in my consciousness' or 'present to my awareness'? The point at issue is just this. We all recognise the terms ⟨Witness⟩, ⟨thoughts⟩, ⟨images⟩, and ⟨sense-data⟩ and know what they denote. If the word ⟨mind⟩ is used only for the first, or first and second, of these, the mental status of the last two, or one, is needlessly prejudiced as one of the proper words can always be used instead of ⟨mind⟩. The mental or other status of sense-data may

[1] We are now postulating the existence of a Pure Ego although Theories I and II do not depend in any way on this assumption.

[2] Although thoughts have no *extension* they have *location* inside the sensed skull.

be decided later after proper enquiry. Price's use of the word leads to confusion: i.e. when he is discussing the Causal Theory he asks why is it necessary to call the table *the* cause of the sense-data. Why not 'the light rays, or the retina, or the brain, or even (perhaps) the mind?' As he has used ⟨mind⟩ before to denote only the Witness (and possibly its associated thought fields: see [*Perception*] page 118) we have here to suppose that processes in the Witness (and possibly its associated thought fields) *cause* sense-data. Just as we saw previously that events in the visual field cannot necessarily be regarded as being caused by events in the s.s.f. in the belief that the latter necessarily is the physical organism, so also, if events in the sensory fields themselves are to be caused by events in the 'mind', then this must not necessarily mean that they are caused by events in the Witness or its thought or even imagery fields: for the mind may be held to include the sensory fields themselves. It seems simpler to say that events in each sensory, thought, and imagery field are causally independent of events in the other fields but each depend separately on events in different parts of the brain, a fact that can be suggested neurologically. For instance, the visual field is affected more by events in the occipital cortex but it is also affected by the parts of the cortex mediating vestibular function.[1]

i.e. _not_ Witness (= mind) ⟫⟶ sensory field

⟫⟶ stands for a relation of causation

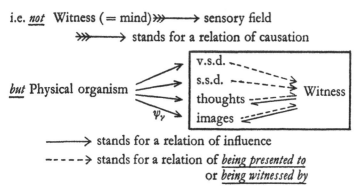

but Physical organism

v.s.d.
s.s.d.
thoughts
images

Witness

ψ_γ

⟶ stands for a relation of influence

----→ stands for a relation of *being presented to*
or *being witnessed by*

Everything inside the rectangle represents the conscious mind of one individual.

[1] Schilder, all works.

On page 80 he gives 'my own body or (in) myself' as containers for 'muscae volitantes, after-images and the spots seen in the field of view when we have a liver attack'. These entities are certainly not in the s.s.f. nor in the Witness. After-images, at least, are surely in the basic *visual field* in which the black or reddish sense-datum we sense when we close our eyes and the stroboscopic patterns are located. And again on page 119 he says:

'If visual and tactual sense-data are processes in the self, the self must be expanded. And if it is expanded, must it not have parts? . . . how can I have parts and yet at the same time possess that unity of consciousness which is necessary to the apprehension of any manifold whatever, whether simultaneous, successive or timeless, and, among other things, to the apprehension of expanses themselves.'

But events may be in the mind without being parts of the Self or Witness. Sense-data are never anywhere except in their own sense-fields, and, if they are in the mind, then the mind *is* expanded and consists of at least two parts, the expanded part (sense and imagery fields) and the unexpanded part—the Self or Witness (and thoughts and feelings). That is not at all the the same as saying that the *Witness* must consist of parts. There is confusion here over the use of the word ⟨self⟩. This may mean the Witness or it may be used in its popular sense to denote *me, my body*, the total organism. For instance:

'Secondly, independence of my will in any case proves nothing. For it is quite compatible with dependence on *myself*, as any dream or hallucination shows. Sense-data might well be caused by psychical process in *me* which had nothing to do with my will, and which were even beyond the reach of introspection' (p. 71—my italics).

Now does ⟨me⟩ here denote my Ego or Witness, or does it denote my total self, my organism? Surely the latter is meant? The argument on pages 70–1 depends entirely on the use of the word ⟨myself⟩. States of *myself* are exemplified by 'my desires, my memories, my interests' (p. 71). Most people regard as their total selves their somatic sensory fields, thought, imagery, and feeling and the Ego or Witness that owns these, and this is the use that Price makes of the term ⟨self⟩ here. But the total organism may be held to include the visual and auditory fields and the physical body as well.

Thus each sense-datum is a part of its own sense-field and each sense-field is a part of the total organism. V.s.d. would then be caused by the non-symbolical representative mechanisms which actually build them up (and the manner of this building is demonstrated by the stroboscopic patterns), and the s.s.d. would be caused by similar mechanisms. These mechanisms may be located in the mind and integrated mechanisms located in the brain. The partial breakdown in their function may be investigated in great detail in cases of brain injury and disease.

Chapter Six

THE STATUS OF MIND IN SHERRINGTON'S PHILOSOPHY

14.   SHERRINGTON in *Man on His Nature*[1] refuses to identify mental experience with electro-chemical events in the brain: nevertheless the mind for him remains 'more ghostly than a ghost. Invisible, intangible, it is a thing not even of outline; it is not a "thing"' (p. 357). He reaches this position through the misuse of the word ⟨mind⟩. He sometimes uses this to denote:

(*a*) the total conscious mind of the Self and its thought, imagery and sense fields;

(*b*) the Self component only together with its thoughts;

(*c*) the sense-fields only;

Thus:

'The mind [*c*] which we experience, if we try to extend our experience into the process of its making, seems to become almost at once unable to be experienced' (p. 307).

'Mind [*c*] providing us with time and space, . . .' (p. 316).

And again (the following passages contain the crux of Sherrington's argument):

'These two concepts, and they are two concepts of one mind

[1] Sir Charles Sherrington, *Man on His Nature*, Cambridge, 1940.

[*a* or *b*], divide, and between them comprise, our world. One of them, the spatial, which we may call the energy-concept, derives by way of the senses. The other, as we saw, is not derived by way of any sense. We saw why. The mind [*b*] has no sense which it can turn inwards so to say upon itself. The idea which mind [*b*] forms of itself lacks extension in space, because sense is required for such extension as a datum, and mind [*b*] does not derive its idea of itself through sense. . . . Extension is what is denied to mind [*a*]' (pp. 348–9).

Note here how the attribute ⟨unextended⟩ relevant to mind (*b*) is illegitimately transferred to mind (*a*) which includes the obviously extended sense-fields, even though Sherrington has said earlier, thus contradicting himself, 'We have, I think, to accept that finite mind is in extended space' (p. 315).

'Between these two, naked mind [*b*] and the perceived world [the sense-fields (mind *c*) identified with the physical world] is there then nothing in common? Together they make up the sum total for us; they are all we have. We called them disparate and incommensurable. Are they then absolutely apart? Can they in no wise be linked together? They have this in common—we have already recognised it—they are both concepts;[1] they both of them are parts of knowledge of one mind [*a*]. They are thus therefore distinguished but are not sundered. Nature in evolving us makes them two parts of the knowledge of one mind [*a*] and that one mind our own' (p. 357).

Thus the sum total of the universe has been reduced to two concepts of a mind which is itself more ghostly than ghost! But the mind itself consists of more than concepts; the conscious mind consists of sense-data of all kinds and images as well. It also seems unwarranted to identify our concepts with physical reality or even with sense-data and images. If we now turn to the context of the phrase quoted above when the mind was reduced to less than a ghost:

'Mind [*b*], for anything perception can compass, goes therefore in our spatial world [*c* identified with the physical world] more ghostly than a ghost. Invisible, intangible, it is a thing not even of outline; it is not a "thing" ' (p. 357).

[1] Here we have a further confusion between the mind (or its parts) and our concept of the mind (or its parts).

We can note that all this is relevant to mind (*b*) but, since Sherrington bases his final account of mind on this, it is wrongly dislocated to mind (*a*).

Sherrington gives the following account of the way in which the subconscious mind may construct consciousness:

'As percept it [the cry of a child in the street] is a complex of certain mental components, a something heard, with "place" "in the street", with time "now", and as to kind or "species" "a human voice", it may be "a child's voice". Whence is all this? The physical sound in the ear was just a physical vibration. How did it generate this mental complex which seems suddenly to invade the mind full-fledged? It cannot have been born full-fledged. It must have gone through a becoming. . . . There would seem therefore to be a grade or grades of mind which we do not experience, as well as the mind which is our mental experience [*c*]' (p. 306).

'It is as though our mind [*c*] were a pool of which the movements on the surface only are what we experience. In the situation we spoke of, the cry was a disturbance gaining entrance somewhere at the bottom of the mental pool. Travelling upwards through the pool it shapes itself and accretes to itself and grows, until reaching the surface it contributes in the form of a percept to the general disturbance obtaining there, and is experienced as part of the mental situation or action which for the time being is experienced' (p. 307).

This analogy may be taken literally, as the sense-fields (most clearly the visual field) are literally surfaces, and the 'pool' is composed of the complex representative mechanisms of the brain and mind whose *function* comprise the subconscious mind. They shape the travelling patterns of their own substance, which 'accrete to themselves and grow' as they pass through to their destination, the sensory fields, where they either form, or at least influence, sense-data in such a way that these latter form the representative picture of the physical world in our consciousness.

EPILOGUE

In an apparently dynamic, incessantly changing world, one of perpetual novelty, the search for things which do not change constitutes one of the principal objectives of science. Philosophers since pre-Socratic times have been rummaging about for the unchanging essence of reality. To-day, that is the job of the scientist.

In topology, as in other branches of mathematics, it takes the form of a search for invariants. Repeatedly, in the course of that search, the necessity arises for abandoning intuition, for transcending imagination. The invariants of 4, 5, 6, and n dimensions are purely conceptual. To fit them into our lives, to find use for them in the laboratory, to shape them for duty in the applied sciences seem impossible. There is nothing in experience to compare them with, not even a dream in which they could play a part.

Nevertheless, what is gathered by the mathematicians, slowly, painfully, bit by bit, in the weird world of beyond-the-make-believe, is in reality a part of the world of everyday, of tides, of cities, and of men, of atoms, of electrons, and of stars. All at once, what came from the land of n dimensions is found useful in the land of three. *Or, perhaps, we discover that after all we live in a land of n dimensions.* It is the reward for the courage and industry, for the fine, untrammelled, poetic, and imaginative sense common to the mathematician, the poet and the philosopher. It is the fulfilment of the vision of science.

KASNER and NEWMAN
from *Mathematics and the Imagination*
(New York, 1940, pp. 297–8) (my italics).

Appendix I

THE EMPIRICAL VERIFICATION
OF THEORIES I AND II

15.   THERE are two more points to clear up from the discussion contained in the first four chapters of this book.

15.1. In 4.22 and 4.331 I stated that it was not impossible, in principle, to confirm the spatial relations postulated by Theory II between sense-data and physical objects by direct observation. That is, it is possible, in principle, to say truthfully 'there's a sense-datum and there's the physical object it belongs to, and I can observe directly that they are spatially related in the manner described in Theory II'. The only reason we cannot do this is that our field of direct observation is only (spatially) three-dimensional, and it would have to be (spatially) four- or more dimensional to get a sense-datum and its related physical object in one field of direct experience so that we could truthfully make the statement given above. That is, we would have to be able to appreciate directly objects bearing higher-dimensional spatial relations to each other.[1] Whitehead's interesting speculations along these lines is given in the Prologue. There is no *a priori* reason why we should not develop the ability to appreciate directly an *n*-dimensional spatial system.

---

[1] This could not be done under Theory I.

15.2. The experimental verification of these new theories of perception (they are cosmological theories as well) depends upon the possibility of detecting the trans-dimensional influences ψ_y and ψ_κ in a physical laboratory. ψ_y may and ψ_κ must cause a considerable disturbance in neuronal activity in the brain very much along the lines suggested by Eccles.[1] ψ_y may be considered to 'scan' the pattern of neuronal excitation in the sensory part of the brain. ψ_y and ψ_κ may be considered to effect an ever-changing pattern of neuronal excitation or facilitation or perhaps only synaptic facilitation in the motor and perhaps the sensory areas. Since the brain is so complex it may never be possible to demonstrate that events there are not determined according to the present laws of physics and that other factors —the 'mind influences' of Eccles—are playing a part. So we must build a model of the brain at a similar degree of 'poise' (Eccles) and see if it behaves as it should according to the predictions we should make using only the present laws of physics. At the same time we can construct the necessary system of mathematical physics which would take into account 'forces' acting upon the physical universe from an origin or location spatially *outside the physical universe* (the meaning of this term ⟨outside⟩ is given in Theories I and II)—for that is how the trans-dimensional influences would appear to a physicist. The general theoretical problem is how can events in one three-dimensional system affect events in another three-dimensional spatial system when the two systems (i) bear higher-dimensional spatial relations to each other, or (ii) bear no spatial relations to each other? The two different systems of mathematical physics based on (i) and (ii) may then lead to different predictions as to the demonstrable effects of 'mind influences' on systems in the physical world. It may be possible to choose between these various systems by experiment and thus gain an empirical confirmation of one of these theories.

[1] J. C. Eccles, *The Neurophysiological Basis of Mind*, Oxford, 1953.

Appendix II

AN ILLUSTRATION OF THEORY II

16.   WE can illustrate Theory IIA as follows. Figure 1 is a picture of a wire model. The wire model itself would represent the three-dimensional geometrical projection of a four-dimensional geometrical figure—the tesseract—just as Figure 2 itself represents the geometrical projection of a three-dimensional figure—the cube—on to a two-dimensional surface. A square may be constructed of four one-dimensional lines set at right angles to each other in a two-dimensional plane. A three-dimensional cube may be constructed from six two-dimensional squares set at right angles to each other in a three-dimensional volume. In an exactly analogous manner a tesseract may be constructed by setting eight three-dimensional cubes at right angles to each other in a four-dimensional space. The wire model of which Figure 1 is a picture bears exactly the same relation to the actual tesseract as the figure drawn in Figure 2 itself bears to the cube.

The eight cubes forming the tesseract are depicted in our wire model by the flat-topped pyramids ABCDA'B'C'D', ABEFA'B'E'F',   CBGFC'B'G'F',   CDGHC'D'G'H', ADHEA'D'H'E', and EFGHE'F'G'H' and by the cubes ABCDEFGH and A'B'C'D'E'F'G'H'. The first six cubes are represented by flat-topped pyramids because of the distortion produced by the geometrical projection, just as four surfaces of the cube (1, 2, 3, 4) are represented in Figure 2 by truncated triangles. The actual wire model pictured in Figure 1 is only the

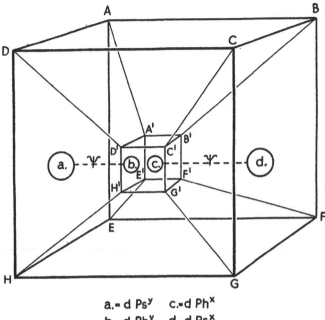

a. = d Ps^y   c. = d Ph^x
b. = d Ph^y   d. = d Ps^x

Fig. 1

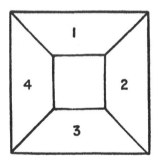

Fig. 2

geometrical projection of the tesseract into three-dimensional space and it is not, it must be emphasised, the tesseract itself. In the tesseract the lines CC', B'C', D'C' and G'C' would all be at right-angles to each other. The tesseract itself cannot of

127

course be drawn or made out of wire models because it is a four-dimensional figure—just as we cannot draw actual cubes on flat pieces of paper.

Now we can use Figure 1 to illustrate what is meant by saying that two three-dimensional spatial systems bear higher-dimensional spatial relations to each other. We can take the cube A'B'C'D'E'F'G'H' to represent the whole physical universe, for there is nothing to prevent us from making the constituent cubes of the tesseract as large as we please. Then the other six cubes (in the actual tesseract it must be remembered) represented in Figure 1 by flat-topped pyramids (i.e. excluding only the cube ABCDEFGH) will represent the entire psychical space systems of six human individuals. If we consider one individual, his brain will occupy a small volume—dPh—inside the cube A'B'C'D'E'F'G'H', and his sense-data and images will occupy a small volume—dPs—inside his psychical space (as in Theory IIA). Each dPs represents Russell's 'private space' of one individual. It is for each of us the familiar space system in which our own visual and somatic sense-data and images are located and extended. Or if we object to this terminology we can say that each dPs is the place where an individual's sense-data and images are. If we consider the individual whose psychical spatial system is represented by the figure CBFGC'B'F'G' then the square C'B'F'G' represents the dimensional interface between his psychical spatial system and the physical spatial system. Whereas the squares CBC'B', CGC'G', BFB'F' and FGF'G' represent the dimensional interfaces between his physical spatial system and those of other people. ψ_y and ψ_x will be wholly spatial causal processes linking dPh and dPs and are represented by dotted lines. In reality the place represented by the bare cube A'B'C'D'E'F'G'H' is filled with stars, planets, seas, brains, trees, fish, etc., while each dPs contains (or 'is filled with' or possibly 'is limited by') sense-data and images.

Figure 1 can also be used to illustrate Theory IIB. In this case the spatial systems represented by the truncated pyramids simply would not exist except for each dPs which would contain, as before, the sense-data and images of the individual. Each dPs would thus not be surrounded by anything, while its sense-data and images would still bear higher-dimensional spatial as well as causal relations to physical objects. Part of ψ in this case connecting dPs with the physical world would consist of non-spatial causal processes.

If we now want to add the psychical spatial systems of more individuals we can merely add as many sets of three axes as we please to form successively higher-dimensional systems. In this figure I have shown the four-dimensional tesseract enclosing the physical universe and the private universes of six individuals. Actually in the $(3m + 3)$ dimensional system it would need a six-dimensional system to enclose the physical universe and the private universe of one individual and it would need a 21-dimensional system to do this in the case of six individuals. But we can only draw projections of four-dimensional figures and not of 21-dimensional figures.

ADDITIONAL NOTES

a. (in introduction) These may be found in *Brit. J. Phil. Sci.*, 1953, **3,** 339–47; 1954, **5,** 120–33; 1956, **6,** 332–5.

b. (in 1.2) A radical behaviourist theory is however presented in (4.4) which may not lead to any logical fallacies although it may be false for other reasons.

c. (in 3.16) An interesting statement of the theory of psycho-neural identity may be found in Polyak, *The Retina*, Chicago, 1941, p. 440.

d. (in 3.162 and 12.6) But see also 4.4.

e. (in 4) All the objections brought forward in this section have been made to me at one time or another by philosophers.

f. (in 4.4) If radical behaviourism were true it would be difficult to see how solipsism could be irrefutable, as it is: that is not to say, of course, that solipsism is true; merely that it is not possible to refute it. It may be argued that the only theory under which *both* solipsism and radical behaviourism could be irrefutable yet false is a theory which accepts the positive existential tenets of both solipsism and radical behaviourism while denying their negative tenets. Thus we can recognise the existence of physical objects, but not physical objects only, and of sense-data, but not of sense-data only.

When I am observing the stroboscopic patterns I am at least as certain that I really am observing this particular pattern—that there is such a pattern in the world and I am looking at it—and that I am not merely undergoing unconscious dispositions to make certain descriptive remarks, as I am certain that there are physical objects: and I am more certain of the existence of these patterns as spatial entities that I can observe than I am certain of the truth of any philosophical theory. But such an opinion must, of course, be personal and could not carry weight against anyone who was prepared to assert the opposite. We could only analyse his reasons for denying the validity of the facts of experience.

g. (in 5.32) It would be better to say here that a single three-dimensional space cannot be literally (geometrically) constructed out of a six-dimensional space and at the same time be all-embracing. No doubt a meaning for 'logical construction' could be found where such an operation could be performed. We can however express all that can usefully be said in this context by talking about geometrical constructions and not logical constructions.

h. (in 7.22) It might be suggested that we need only a seven-dimensional space for our purpose—i.e. a three-dimensional physical space plus a number of three-dimensional sensible subsections of a common four-dimensional space in which all minds were 'stacked', just as we can stack as many planes as we wish in a cube. However this would mean that physical space could only be contiguous with two sensible spaces, each of which would separate physical space from the rest of the 'stack': whereas it would seem preferable that physical space should be contiguous with each and every sensible space as it is in the $(3m + 3)$-dimensional model. But it may be that there are a number of possible systems and this may offer a field for research for a geometer.

k (in 10.15) Among many other examples from experimental psychology are all forms of apparent movement, and the phenomena described by Pulfrich, Werner, and Ames.

m. (in 10.222) The latest experimental work indicates that these phenomena are predominantly of cerebral origin.

n. (in 12.81) Whorf, like most innovators carried his ideas somewhat to excess, but his main ideas seem sensible enough.

ab. (in 3.1) The argument given in (3.1) is meant to show that material objects cannot be directly observed for reasons hinging on the finite velocity of light. This may be put as follows. The entity which may be observed to bear spatial relations to an after-sensation of the kind described in (2.1) cannot be identical with the material thing which a naïve realist would say that it *was*, for the reason that the two entities are at opposite ends of a causal chain and, at any particular instant of time, have different temporal co-ordinates relative to any one set of spatio-temporal axes. In the perception of a star the little twinkly object that is *seen* (on a naïve realist theory) cannot be identical with the material object, for the latter is very much in the *future* relative to the former—that is, they have different temporal co-ordinates. This argument may be developed as follows:

Let us imagine two observers on two planets. The planets are not in relative motion and are separated by a distance of *w* light-years. Observer *a* on planet A directs an (extremely powerful) telescope at planet B and sees observer *b* gazing up his (equally powerful) telescope in his direction. Will *b*, we can ask, likewise see *a* gazing at him? The answer is that he would not. He will see planet A 2*w* years before *a* directs his telescope at B on the occasion described above. Let us say that *w* is 10 and that when *a* directs his telescope at B he is 21 years old. Therefore *b* will see *a* as a baby 1 year old. Now the theory of naïve realism states that it is always literally the material object itself that we sense in a non-hallucinatory perception. Therefore the real material man *a* is looking at and seeing the real material man *b*. Similarly the theory must hold that the real material man *b* is, while *a* is watching *him*, in turn watching (and seeing) the real material baby *a*, aged 1. For we cannot claim that any man's frame of reference is any more absolute than any other man's. Therefore, on the occasion that *a* directs his telescope at B described above, *a* must have two material bodies, one of which is seeing *b* and the other is being seen by *b* while *b* is being seen by *a*. In a similar manner *a* can be shown to have any number of material bodies depending on how many observers in other parts of the universe could logically observe him. For it must be said that each observer is seeing a real material object and each observer will, if located at different distances away, see *a*'s body at different periods in its history. Consider further that while *b* is observing *a* as a one-year-old baby he (*b*) will not be aware that the 21-year-old *a* is actually watching him. In an exactly similar manner may not an older *b* be observing the 21-

year-old *a* while *a* is watching the younger *b*? And the older *b* in turn may be observed by a yet older *a*, and so we start on a regress the number of terms of which is limited only by the longevity of *a* and *b*? To make this clearer suppose that *a* and *b* are the same age and consider *a* aged 61. He looks through his telescope at *b* and sees the 51-year-old *b* looking through *his* telescope and seeing the 41-year-old *a*, who, as it happens, is looking through his telescope and seeing the 31-year-old *b*, who . . . and so on and so on. If the theory of naïve realism is true all these *a*'s and *b*'s are equally real material objects. For if one man sees another it is the material object (man) that he sees.

By varying *w* as we may we find that material objects throughout the universe must be equally real at all 'instants' in their histories. That is to say we are postulating a Hinton universe; i.e. that the material world is composed not of three-dimensional solids enduring in time, existing only in the 'present' with no concrete reality in the future or in the past, but of four-dimensional solids extended into the spatial past and spatial future. For *b* as *a* sees him is certainly spatially extended and is equally certainly in *a*'s past as we commonly understand 'past'. The fact of the finite velocity of light combined with the postulate that, in perception, we observe material objects themselves directly *necessitates* the spatialisation of time and the postulation of a Hinton universe. Ordinarily we suppose that our bodies, as well as other material things, of *x* years ago no longer exist as such but that they only exist 'now'. We think that the body that existed *x* years ago has *changed* into my body that I can feel and see 'now'. But if naïve realism is true we must say that our infant bodies exist still for it is logically possible that they may be seen by any *b* and it is also logically possible that we can see *b* seeing them. This is so because naïve realism has *two* criteria (but not only two criteria) for the existence of human bodies during any one short period of time—*to see* and *to be seen*.

It may however be claimed that what is seen does not necessarily exist. But if this argument is brought in to account for the perception of distant objects we must say that nothing that we see exists for all visual perception is mediated by light the velocity of which is finite (to say nothing of the sluggardly impulses in the optic nerve). But this is surely not the position

that the naïve realist set out to defend? If I say that I am seeing
the non-existent past state of a material thing this object must
also have a 'present' state otherwise there would not be any
non-existent past state of the object for me to see in, say, eight
minutes' time. This present state of the object I do not see and
thus the basic premiss of naïve realism is refuted. This argument can also be stated as follows: 'For *x* to be a material thing
it is necessary for it to exist. Therefore we do not see material
things for what we see does not exist.' Furthermore if nothing
that we see (or hear or touch—the velocity of sound waves and
of the impulses in somatic sensory nerves is also finite) exists
what then does exist? It would surely be equally unsatisfactory
to answer 'material things but not when we see them' (for this
refutes naïve realism) and 'only thoughts and images' (for this
is worse than solipsism).

It can be argued that the only defence open to the naïve
realist is to postulate a Hinton universe for this is the only universe in which past objects that may be seen really do still exist.
However a Hinton universe entails certain consequences that
I am sure that most naïve realists would be most unwilling to
accept. For the Hinton universe *necessitates* a dualist theory of
mind and it is precisely to escape from such a theory that many
philosophers support naïve realism. In the physical Hinton universe there is nothing whatever to indicate any 'now' of time
and moreover there can be no movement of objects. Material
things, including human bodies and brains, merely extend in
their complex frozen four-dimensional shapes from the beginning to the end of time. There is no intrinsic movement in such
a universe. It is necessary to introduce an extraneous 'observer'
the movement of whose field of observation *past* the four-
dimensional objects produces both the shifting 'now' of time
and the appearance of moving three-dimensional material objects which are 'really' successive cross-sections of the four-
dimensional solids.

In the examples given above we took observers separated by
a great distance to emphasize the paradox. But the argument
holds equally well for observers any distance apart. Observer *a*
could as well be on Earth and observer *b* on the moon. In which
case no very startling advance in telescope technology and inter-

planetary travel may render the observations described above empirically as well as logically possible. Observer *b* can also be replaced by an immense mirror or system of prisms. In which case we could be said to see the previous states of our own bodies, or, as we should have to say, our previous bodies.

So to review the situation we have reached. In the common usage of language there is no warrant to challenge any commonly accepted perceptual statements such as 'I see a cow'. But in giving a scientific account of perception we can either deny the occurrence of experiential events and take up the radical behaviourist theory; or, if we accept the occurrence of experiential events, we must distinguish between *perceiving material objects*, which necessitates the whole causal chain—object-light-retina-brain-experiential event together with the sensing of the latter, and *sensing sensible objects* (sense-data) which may either be a *part* of perceiving material objects, or it may not as in the case of hallucinations. Naïve realism makes the mistake of *identifying* perceiving material objects with sensing sensible objects and calling both seeing objects, whereas only the former can properly be called *seeing* material objects. The part-whole relation between sensing and perceiving is the source of most of the muddle.

I am most grateful to Professor C. D. Broad who very kindly read a condensation of the argument and suggested the point discussed in note *h*, and to James Thomson and Seymour Papert whose advice has enabled me to avoid some serious mistakes.

INDEX

Index

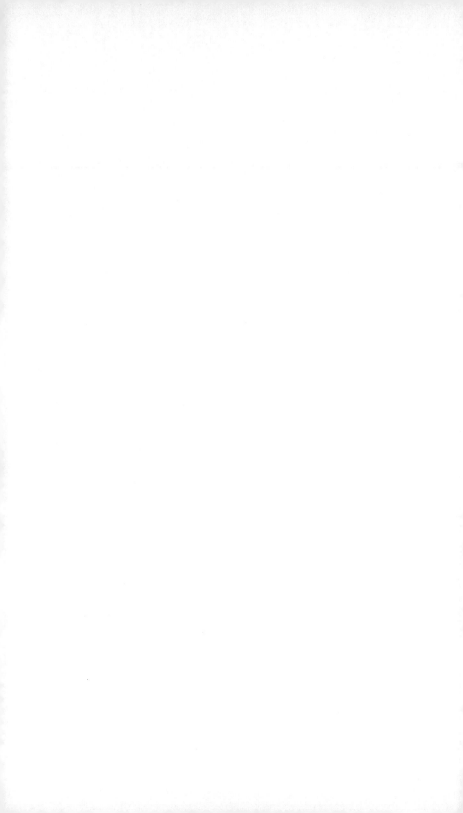